Andrew,
Thank You For T⟨...⟩

Journey
to a
New You

A Transformational Guide to
Discovering Your Inner Strengths

Sharon D. Meadows

SHARON D. MEADOWS

Andrew,

Thank You For Being A Friend!

ISBN: 0989322505

ISBN 13: 9780989322508

Library of Congress Control Number: 2013907784

J'Lyn Star Publishing, Houston, TX

Important Medical Disclaimer

Disclaimer for <u>Journey to a New You: A Transformational Guide to Discovering Your Inner Strengths</u>

J'LYN STAR PUBLISHING IS PROVIDING *JOURNEY TO A NEW YOU: A TRANSFOR-MATIONAL GUIDE TO DISCOVERING YOUR INNER STRENGTHS* (HEREAFTER REFERRED TO AS "BOOK") AND IT'S CONTENTS ON AN "AS IS" BASIS AND MAKES NO REPRESEN-TATIONS OR WARRANTIES OF ANY KIND WITH RESPECT TO THIS BOOK OR ITS CON-TENTS. J'LYN STAR PUBLISHING DISCLAIMS ALL REPRESENTATIONS AND WARRAN-TIES FOR MERCHANTABILITY AND FITNESS FOR A PARTICULAR PURPOSE.

The statements made regarding meal plans have not been evaluated by the US Food and Drug Administration. They are not intended to diagnose, treat, cure, or prevent any condition or disease. Please consult with your physician or health care provider regarding the suggestions and recommendations made within this book.

Except as specifically stated in this book, Sharon D. Meadows, J'Lyn Star Publishing, contributors, or other representatives will not be liable for damages arising from or in connection with the use of this book. This is a comprehensive limitation of liability that applies to all damages of any kind, including (without limitation) compensatory damages; direct, indirect, or consequential damages; loss of data, income, or profit; loss of or damage to property; and claims of third parties.

This book provides content related to topics on nutrition and fitness. As such, use of this book implies your acceptance of the terms described herein.

You understand that the author is not a licensed health care professional. You understand that this book is provided to you without a health examination and without prior discussion of your current health condition. You understand that in no way will this book provide medical advice and that no medical advice is contained within this book or the content provided.

You understand that this book is not intended as a substitute for consultation with a licensed health care provider such as your physician. Before beginning any weight loss program or change of your nutrition regimen, you should consult with your physician or other licensed health care provider to ensure that you are in good health and that the recommendations contained in this book will not cause any harm to you.

If you experience any unusual symptoms after following any information in this book, you will stop performing the advice of this book and consult with your health care provider immediately.

You understand that the information and content of this book should not be used to diagnose a health problem or disease, or to determine any health-related treatment program, including weight loss, diet, or exercise.

You understand that there are risks with engaging in any activity described in this book. Any action you take implies that you assume all risks, known and unknown, inherent to exercises, workout programs, nutrition programs, physical changes, and/or injuries that may result from the actions that you take.

You hereby release Sharon D. Meadows and J'Lyn Star Publishing from any liability related to this book to the fullest extent permitted by law. This includes any damages, costs, or losses of any nature arising from the use of this book and information provided by this book, including direct, consequential, special, punitive, or incidental damages, even if Sharon D. Meadows or J'Lyn Star Publishing have been advised of the possibility of such damages.

Your use of this book confirms your agreement to the above terms and conditions. If you do not agree, you will not utilize this book and will request a full refund within the time frame specified in your contract of sale.

Dedications

Most important, to God, the one who makes all things possible. To him, I lift up praise and humble gratitude. Thank you.

To Mom and Grandma Edith, thank you for always believing in me, and for always being the pillars that supported my dreams. Grandma Edith, I know you are watching from above, proud of me.

To Jaylyn and Jayda, my daughters, thank you for giving me sunshine on cloudy days. You have been the best part of my life. Jaylyn, you are greatly missed and will forever live in my heart.

To Nicholas, my brother, thank you for your continuous support along the way.

To Nike Fashokun, your support, love and friendship have been paramount in my development as a woman, writer, and speaker. Thank you for always being there, holding my hand every step of the way.

To Barbara Curtis, thank you for being my friend, supporter, and mentor in the down season; now that the season has shifted, I hope that you are proud.

To Surrenda Jones, my sister in Christ, thank you for cheering from the sidelines and being a part of the "dream" team; and may together we always dream BIG!

To Daniel Adeyemo, thank you for igniting the fire within me to write and for believing I could do it.

Contents

Introduction

S everal months ago, a friend invited me to attend an event at the Los Angeles Convention Center that was sponsored by Oprah Winfrey. It was called "O You!" and it inspired all in attendance to learn to live their best lives.

Several of the Oprah experts spent the day sharing insightful wisdom that could be applied to various aspects of life. I had the pleasure to hear Dr. Laura Berman, Martha Beck, Gayle King, Peter Walsh, Dr. Phil McGraw, Suze Orman, and Iyanla Vanzant speak, and even Oprah blessed us with her infinite wisdom. It was truly an extraordinary experience.

Of all the entertaining stories that were shared that day, one really lingered in my mind long after the event concluded. It was a story told by Dr. Phil about a time when Oprah had invited him to spend time with her and a few of her friends at a girls' retreat.

Dr. Phil said the ladies wanted him in attendance for one reason and one reason only: they wanted him to tell them why they were fat. He said they all sat around with notepads and pens in hand waiting to hear his profound insightful response. Oprah and her friends truly believed that Dr. Phil had the answer they so desperately wanted to hear.

Dr. Phil said he was open and honest when he provided his answer to the ladies. If you have ever seen Dr. Phil, the one thing that you and I can agree on without a doubt is that he is direct. He told Oprah and her friends what he thought the reason was, and he didn't hold back. Dr. Phil responded to the ladies by saying, "You are fat because you want to be fat, simple as that."

Now, I don't know if I heard anything that Dr. Phil said beyond that point. That one statement alone stopped me in my tracks and made me think, could he be right? Are people fat because they want to be fat?

I took a moment to digest his response. I began to ponder the thought, actually reflecting on my own life and the times I had been overweight. During my life, I have been fat—and I can assure you that I did not want to be.

I don't personally know Oprah, but I would assume that she has never strived to be fat. Being a fan of Oprah, I am well aware that Oprah has invested time, energy, and effort into actually being the total opposite of fat.

On the other hand, I could understand the point Dr. Phil was attempting to drive home. In my mind, I assume, what he was conveying was that losing weight is a personal choice—and he is correct, it is. The challenge is that once you decide you actually want to lose the weight, the course of action that you partake will lead you to a journey. It takes more than just desiring to lose weight; you must make a choice.

If you are like me, you have taken the journey multiple times in life. Once you reach success, you feel in control and you feel empowered; you are on top of the world. When faced with an unwelcome setback you feel defeated, disappointed, and discouraged—the feelings of failure.

One setback that I have experienced personally, as have others close to me, is the inability to avoid falling off course for one reason or another. Once this occurs, getting back on track can sometimes seem impossible.

Falling off track generally occurs when there is a lack of understanding that the distance you travel on this journey is not the destination. The final destination on this journey is a permanent lifestyle change. The journey to healthier eating does not end when you reach a goal (i.e., your target weight). This journey will result in a long-term lifestyle change that will bring about new changes in your eating habits. To sustain your results, you will be required to commit to these changes, whatever they may be, for the rest of your life.

If you haven't fully grasped the lifelong commitment this journey will require then think of it as you would marriage. Marriage is a lifelong commitment—that is, till death do you part. So, what does marriage require? It requires commitment, loyalty, honesty, and trust, just to name a few things. When you think of your eating habits, ask yourself: Are you committed, loyal, honest, and trustworthy when it comes to food? Or do you find yourself cheating?

Many people would never cheat on their spouses, yet they cheat themselves daily by misbehaving with food. Why is it easier to live by one set of principles for one aspect in your life and more difficult to apply those same principles in other areas? Most of us are guilty of this, including me.

When thinking back to the comment that Dr. Phil made to Oprah and her friends, I was forced to ask myself, is anyone fat because they truly want to be that way? Honestly, I doubt it. Are people overweight, obese, or just plain not satisfied with their appearance? Yes, of course, some people are, and their reasons are many.

Dr. Phil's perception on weight control to me is clear. He is suggesting that if you are fat and you don't like it, then you should chose to do something about it. I agree with him on this matter wholeheartedly.

At the same time, I believe the old adage holds true: it's easier said than done. As with most difficult things in our life, bringing about change is not that easy.

Changing is easier said than done, but not impossible. So how do you bring about change? I know the way, I go the way daily, and I can show you the way. Allow me to be your guide on a journey where there is no true final destination. I will travel alongside you as your friend as you embark on changes to make a lifelong commitment. I will get you to where you want to be.

The majority of the journey will be affected by your thoughts, actions, feelings, and emotions. All of these things will determine your success or lack thereof. So where does this journey begin? It begins with a simple question. Ask yourself today, what's in it for me? Take the time to honestly answer this question, and we shall go on from there.

CHAPTER I

Breaking Bad Habits

I recently uncovered an interesting concept while reading a fitness magazine. The article suggested that it takes approximately twenty-one days to change a bad habit. Supposedly a bad habit is any negative behavior that you frequently engage in. The upside to this is that all of us have control over our habits, be they good or bad.

Through willpower and determination you can correct any habit that you have ever established in your life. I am sure that you and I are both guilty of having a few bad habits. When it comes to food, stop for a moment and think about some of your current bad habits.

One day while I was sitting at Starbucks, I stared out the window and thought about some of my own bad habits. I thought back through the many years and tried to identify previous bad habits that I have been able to correct. You and I both actually have the ability to correct any habits they we may have developed in any areas of our lives.

As I sat staring out the window, one bad habit that popped into my mind had nothing to do with my eating behavior. Over a period of time, I was able to follow a few simple concepts to break this particular habit. I had unknowingly established a bad habit of kicking off my shoes immediately after walking in the front door of my home. I did it every single day. I can honestly say I was not completely aware of my actions. I realized that nearly every single pair of shoes that I owned were literally spread from one angle of my foyer to the next. When I had visitors over, it was rather embarrassing. Before long I began to make excuses as to why my foyer was the designated storage space for all of the shoes that I owned.

I would first apologize for the untidiness that my shoes created. Then I would cleverly create excuses as to why my shoes were scattered all about the foyer. Inside I would feel utter embarrassment as I sensed I was being secretly judged by others. All the while, I would never do anything to make a decision to clean up my pile of shoes. Even though I didn't like it, I chose to do nothing about it. I became comfortable with my unpleasant feelings about the scattered shoes, and I soon began to accept those feelings.

Deep down, I felt that I honestly didn't like the appearance of the shoes being scattered throughout the foyer. I didn't like the judgment that I thought visitors were passing when they saw the shoes. I would rationalize and negotiate the excuses in my mind, allowing myself to lessen the guilt that I felt.

Yet somehow my own disapproval as well as my perceived disapproval from others did not have enough impact on me to make a change, even though I knew that I desperately needed to.

I would actually think about organizing my shoes, but I would not put any action behind my thoughts. On rare occasions, I would talk about how I planned to take action to get more organized. I would imagine details on how I planned to get started. Yet, with no clear plan of action, I did nothing. The end result was that day after day the shoes remained in disarray in my home. I found myself constantly talking about making changes. The truth is, thought with no action will only allow you to continue to engage in the same bad behavior as before. Without putting forth any plan of action, I made absolutely no change in my behavior.

Here is the funny thing about excuses: sometimes they actually don't make any sense even though you try to convince yourself otherwise. In my opinion, excuses are just clever ways of avoiding the truth.

No matter what excuses I created in my mind, my truth and reality still existed. The truth was that I had a cluttered array of shoes scattered throughout my foyer, and I had chosen to take no clear action to rectify the problem. The only action I had actually taken was to make excuses for myself to continue what was clearly a bad habit.

If I thought long and hard enough, I could probably even pinpoint when I started kicking my shoes off in the foyer. I was pretty sure it had been going on for many years. Many bad habits that you or I may have didn't just start yesterday. A habit, after all, has to be established. It's a repetitive behavior, something you do over and over again with consistency. Once you accept a bad behavior, you feel more comfortable continuing to engage in it, thereby repeating it.

For me, the turning point was one afternoon while at the home of a friend; I caught a glimpse of her closet. When I walked in, I couldn't believe my eyes. She had not only organized each and every pair of shoes that she owned on the shelves but had actually put them in individual clear containers. On the outside of each container was a Polaroid picture of the shoe. This conveniently provided her a way to easily identify the shoe without actually opening the container.

I left my friend's home that afternoon with one thought in mind. In fact, my friend had given me a few great suggestions as to how to get started. The one thought I had was, the first thing the next morning I would organize my shoes.

Now, I knew that I honestly had no intention of going to the extent that my friend had gone—there was no way, it would be far too time-consuming for me. What I did know was that I would need to actually put forth some type of effort to change my current behavior. Sometimes seeing someone who is successful in an area in which you lack discipline is all the motivation you need. I am no exception to this rule; it was, after all, my friend's motivation that gave birth to a change in my own behavior.

The next day, the first item on my to-do list was to come up with my own personalized plan to organize my shoes. I sat down and figured out what I really would be comfortable with, and I decided that I did actually want the shoes near the front door. I didn't want a plan that would be so off-base for me that it would only last temporarily. I also knew that I needed the change to be reasonable in order for it to be sustainable; otherwise I would be setting myself up for failure.

Trying to take the approach that my friend had taken would have only resulted in me eventually returning to my previous behavior. I needed something that was more realistic and suitable for me.

The next day, as I was casually strolling through Bed Bath & Beyond I saw a shoe organizer. Immediately I knew it would work for me and my needs. I purchased it, put it together, and placed it near the staircase, out of plain view. Although the shoes were still in the foyer, they were now neatly organized and arranged in a way that I could maintain and that was not noticeable to my visitors.

I felt extremely proud of myself for making the change. A sense of accomplishment began to motivate me, and because I had taken an approach that I could actually maintain, I was able to make the change long-term. It's been a year since I made the change, and I have not reverted back to my old bad behavior.

If you are scratching your head by now, wondering what the heck shoes being scattered throughout the foyer have to do with me giving practical insight on helping you to lose weight, then good, I have your attention.

Aside from me sharing with you that I am not the most organized person, I have just illustrated a simple concept that contained a few key components:

#1. Identifying an established bad habit

#2. Making excuses to continue the bad habit

#3. Rationalizing and negotiating bad behavior

#4. Dissatisfaction with the behavior causing the bad habit

#5. Taking no corrective actions to stop the bad habit

#6. Creating an action plan to stop the bad habit

#7. Putting intentional action to the plan

#8. Successful elimination of the bad habit

I chose the illustration of the shoes to demonstrate that a bad habit can be eliminated with the right plan of action regardless of what that habit may be. I could have used smoking, biting your finger nails, or drinking too much caffeine—you get the point.

It is my belief that for many people their unhealthy eating habits have evolved from what started as an innocent bad habit. Today, take a step toward breaking your bad eating habits by vowing to yourself to make a conscious change.

The key to achieving success is to start with the right plan of action and to exercise discipline and self-control. I cannot promise you that you will break your bad eating habits and develop healthier ones within twenty-one days. The success that you experience will solely depend on you and your level of commitment and dedication.

According to a recent study at the University College of London, the average time it takes a person to form a new habit is sixty-six days. This means that you will need to begin making changes by taking small and deliberate steps. More important than making the changes you need to make, you will need to be patient with yourself by being understanding and forgiving of yourself as you implement the changes.

Please remember that you are not on this journey alone. I have successfully taken the journey, and I will take the journey with you, every single step of the way. During the course of this book, I will help you to identify the root cause of bad eating habits that you have developed and to work on actions to replace or correct those behaviors.

I will be your friend, leader, personal coach, and source of support with every turn of each page. I will be with you along the entire journey, and will be standing with you as you overcome each of your struggles to celebrate your victories and successes.

I am totally committed to helping you develop long-term solutions that you can implement to create healthier eating habits that will leave you looking and feeling great!

CHAPTER 2

The Naked Truth

Weeks after giving birth to my daughter, Jayda, I began to take inventory on my body. I was reminded daily of the extra weight. It was continuously a part of my thought processes, day in and day out.

I soon began to practice certain techniques with my clothing that would allow me to easily camouflage the extra pounds. At the end of the day, I was faced with the truth, and it wasn't going away easily. Once I shed my clothes down to the bare minimum, my reality was greatly exposed; I was no longer able to hide it.

Each day after I showered, I would stand in the mirror and quickly dry myself to avoid catching a glimpse of the truth. I knew if I actually looked, I wouldn't like the image that was looking back at me. I was convincing myself that if I didn't look at my body I could avoid having any negative feelings about my appearance. Honestly, I don't know who I thought I was fooling.

How many different times in your own life can you think of situations in which you have tried to ignore the truth by not facing it head-on? I'm here to tell you that trying to ignore the truth by avoiding it is a waste of time. The truth doesn't change just because you don't face it; it is indeed still there.

Personally, I have ignored the truth more times than I care to remember. I don't just mean when it came to my weight, either. For example, years ago I realized I was extremely unhappy in my marriage. Instead of facing the truth and dealing with my immeasurable misery, I would camouflage it, cover it up, and conceal it by any means necessary.

The unfortunate problem with concealing the truth is that sooner or later you will have to face it. In my own experience, the longer that I continued to sweep my truth under the rug, the more devastating the face-to-face confrontation would tend to be.

When I think about facing the truth when it comes to weight gain, I think of many words to describe why someone may fear his or her own personal truth. I will use myself as an example. When I would look in the mirror, the words that would come to my mind were words such as *pain*, *despair*, *disgust*, and *disappointment*, just to name a few. These negative words would then manifest into negative thoughts about myself. To avoid these negative feelings I would avoid looking in the mirror.

Negative feelings that sometimes accompany the truth are feelings of embarrassment, guilt, shame—the list can go on and on. It is totally understandable to me as to why anyone would shy away from the truth if the truth is not desirable. However, facing the truth forces uncomfortable or difficult parts in life to become more real, to no longer be swept under the rug or overlooked.

I have learned that the times when I have experienced the most peace and joy have been those times when I have been truly authentic, embracing my truth. There is indeed a benefit in facing the truth: with it comes a sense of freedom. And freedom brings a sense of relief, resulting in a sense of internal acceptance and peace.

Confronting the truth also provides the confronter with the ability to recognize that a problem actually exists, and it allows room to create change to foster growth. Creating change requires you to face the truth and then accept it. Understanding the underlying causes of a problem is imperative. If you don't fully understand a problem, then it is impossible to demonstrate the ability to fix it.

Now, back to my former marriage. During the course of seven years, I would sit on my sofa and cry endlessly. The thought racing through my mind during the crying bouts was, why doesn't this man want me to be happy? I honestly had no idea.

On the outside, to others, I maintained the appearance that my marriage was a happy one. On the inside, the truth was far from marital bliss. Now, don't get me wrong, I am fully aware that all marriages have struggles and that there is no perfect marriage. However, a marital union should be healthy, and mine was far from healthy. Each day I continued to slog through it, never facing the truth—*my* truth. My real truth was that my marriage was making me miserable and it was coming to an end.

I can recall coming home after work one day and sitting in the driveway. I was feeling as though I just didn't want to get out of the car. I just didn't want to go in the house and face it, face *him*. Do you recall that I said when we don't like our truth, we try to avoid it? I am no exception to these types of feelings and I totally understand why someone may run from the truth. I could avoid the truth as long as I wanted, but eventually I would be forced to face it. Eventually, I knew that I would have to go in the house; there was no way around it.

I could sit in the car as long as I wanted, but my truth still remained on the opposite side of the door. I had a husband in the house and he caused me to feel miserable. That was my truth, whether I liked it or not.

The day that I actually made the decision to file for divorce, it was as if a huge burden had been lifted from my shoulders. I felt that I could finally breathe. I can remember lying in bed, exhaling slowly, and although my heart was breaking inside, I still had a huge sense of relief. I am not glamorizing divorce by any means, and for me it was a last resort. The point is, once I faced my truth I was unequivocally set free.

Looking back on my marriage, I realized a few things. If I had faced the truth early on and not tried to avoid it, I could have actually addressed the problems and found a feasible solution. This could have possibly resulted in a more desirable outcome, avoiding divorce altogether.

The interesting thing about insight is that you unfortunately don't have it until you look back at an experience in retrospect. Insight is, without a doubt, the hindsight of experience. Honestly, my ability to face the truth would have allowed me to identify the problem areas and face them head-on. How can you find a solution to correct a problem when you have no clear understanding of what the problem actually is? The fact is, you can't.

You have to be honest and look at a problem face-to-face to fix it even if it is painful, scary, embarrassing or negative in any other way that comes to mind. When you are face-to-face with a truth that you do not desire, the best question you can ask yourself is, how did I get here?

If you are honest in answering this question, then I believe you are on the road to reshaping the truth into something that you will welcome and embrace.

Take a moment to ask yourself what your truth is right now. On this journey, there is no ridicule, judgment, shame, or blame. As your friend, I will support you in discovering your truth regarding food— whatever that truth may be.

Today, begin to face your truth. Look in the mirror and ask the question, how did I get here? Then give life to your truth by writing it down. List all the truths that you can identify to answer the question of how you arrived at this place. You will not remain here, but you need first to understand how you arrived here.

Truth #1 _____

Truth #2 _____

Truth #3 _____

Truth #4 _____

Truth #5 _____

Truth #6 _____

While writing this book, I decided to interview my friend Judith. She had made a conscious decision to lose weight, so I thought she was an ideal candidate who could provide a fresh perspective. Judith gained forty pounds over the previous two years. She and I sat and tried to pinpoint the cause of her weight gain. I asked Judith to identify events, if any, which had occurred in her life over the previous two years.

She began by telling my about a new job that she had decided to take that had resulted in overwhelming stress for her. She then said she had left that job and stepped out on faith to start her own accounting firm.

During the same month she also received an approval letter from the CPA board qualifying her to take the CPA exam. A few months later her daughter left home and went off to college.

She told me none of the events were bad things, aside from the stressful job that she had taken during that time; she said all the events were good things. Over the previous two years, she had actually been excited by everything that was going on in her life. As she and I probed the events from the previous two years, we were able to identify that change in her life is a trigger.

Judith quickly began to realize that any type of change, good or bad, would send her eating habits into a reckless tailspin, causing her to pack on unwanted pounds.

As we sat and talked about the events that had occurred in her life we were able to unravel many important factors. Judith revealed to me that she loves structure; she has to have it. Without structure, she feels lost, with no direction. Judith told me that she was most effective if she could live her life by a checklist. She said she needed to know what to expect each hour of the day. Otherwise, the lack of direction caused major disruption in her daily activities.

Even though she was excited about the new business venture, she said it had come with much uncertainty. She was forced to engage new clients, many of whom she did not know. The new unfamiliarity of not personally knowing her clients created a high level of stress.

Although the approval letter from the CPA board brought her great joy, there was a level of stress that came with it. Judith knew she was going to need to study and prepare for the exam. The preparation time needed to study was outside her daily routine. With that study time being outside her norm, it was nearly impossible for her to factor it in. The end result was that she was unprepared when the time arrived to take the exam.

Judith was also accustomed to having lots of activities with her daughter on her daily schedule. These activities ranged from sports to school activities to social events. When her daughter left, she felt a void in her life. Judith was overwhelmed by all of the free time, and she had no idea what to do with it or how to manage it.

When these changes started occurring, she quickly began to lose focus. The anxiety and fear that she was experiencing caused her to have many sleepless nights. She found herself sluggish each morning, and to give herself a boost she began indulging in junk food. Bad idea!

On most days she thought the sugar rush would give her a quick pick-me-up. Judith also noticed that the lack of focus and structure in her life caused her to forget to eat proper meals like lunch or dinner— sometimes both. By forgetting to eat and skipping meals, she was slowing down her metabolism, thereby forcing her body into storage mode. She wasn't overeating, but she also wasn't losing any weight.

By the end of the interview, we were able to obtain some level of clarity pertaining to her problem areas. Judith shared with me that she was beginning to feel more in control of her situation. By identifying her problem areas, we could then pinpoint the trigger that caused her to engage in her bad habit of eating sweets and junk food. Her trigger clearly was change; she now knew what she needed to do when faced with change, be it good or bad. Judith's sense of being in control was clearly a result of her ability to understand the relationship between triggers and problem areas.

The solution to Judith's problem was not a simple one, but it was doable. I suggested that she be aware of her triggers when change is happening in her life and that she stop to become aware of the change. She can then move on slowly, with direction and purpose, prepared for a setback in her eating habits.

Judith will need to be resilient in the journey to handle any types of change that come her way. She will need to be able to allow changes to occur in her life while preventing herself from being knocked off course. Being aware of your triggers puts you in control. Being in control of your situation prevents you from making bad choices that may ultimately catch you off guard, thereby knocking you off track. When a trigger comes your way, your awareness will decrease your chances of it resulting in a setback.

As you begin your journey, be bold and look your truth in the face, whatever that truth may be. Knowing how you arrived at this place is instrumental in your ability to move away from this place. Remember, it doesn't matter where you are, but *how you got here* does matter.

To move forward with change you must really understand your problem areas. To understand your problem areas, you must identify the triggers related to them. List the triggers associated with each problem area you can think of. After you have identified the problem areas and triggers, identify alternatives with which to counter each trigger.

Problem Triggers   **Problem Area**   **Alternatives**

By identifying your problem areas, you just took a major step toward making a positive change in your lifestyle. Knowing your problem areas and your triggers will empower you to be able to counter setbacks before they actually occur. You just took the first step in dealing with your truth, and that took a great deal of courage! Congratulations!

If you are having difficulty determining what your problem areas and triggers are, here are a few examples that might help generate your own ideas.

• **Problem Triggers:**	Large portions;	Coffee with creamer;	Eating too much bread
• **Problem Area:**	Portion control;	Daily habit;	Bread before meals
• **Alternatives:**	Smaller portions;	Green tea;	Avoiding bread before meals

There are no right or wrong answers for this exercise. The focus should be on getting a handle on your problem areas by understanding the root cause of the problems. If you are unable to identify the trigger associated with the problem area then you will be less likely to bring a positive change to your current behavior.

Over the course of this journey, you will be working toward eliminating problem areas by avoiding triggers. For me, portion control was a problem area. The behavioral change that I had to make was to be fully aware of the portion sizes that I consumed with each meal. I discovered that the only way to change my behavior in order to eliminate the problem was to be more deliberate and intentional with the amount of food I consumed for each meal.

Making a lifestyle change requires commitment, discipline, and effort. To achieve the results that you desire, you will have to avow to yourself that you are totally committed to the journey. Start the journey by telling yourself that you are making a pledge to lose weight and to eat healthier. Now give life to your thoughts and speak your pledge aloud.

The next thing that you will need on your journey is discipline. Don't worry; I know firsthand how difficult this one is. You will succeed in this area with no problem. In chapter 6 you will work on techniques to improve and increase your disciplinary skills. The last component that will be needed is effort. Losing weight and eating healthy food takes work. The key is in knowing that you have total control in this area. This means that your results will reflect the investment that you are willing to make in yourself. You will have total control over the results that you achieve, and it will be based on the amount of effort that you are willing to apply. Exercising discipline may not seem pleasant at times; in some cases it can actually be painful. Discipline produces rewards for those who have been trained by it. Understand that the more effort you apply toward being disciplined, the greater your reward.

Let's add a little more perspective. After my divorce, dating was extremely difficult. I was starting from scratch with romance. I was a little overwhelmed at the thought of meeting new people, spending time with them, and getting to know them. Honestly, I simply just wanted to meet someone I liked, and then catapult at full speed into a relationship. I now realize this was not the best way of thinking.

I eventually met a young man I liked, and after three dates I decided, OK, this is the one. Initially he was very responsive in wanting to see me, but when I went at full speed he started to back away. Actually, he *ran* away! I asked a male friend if he could possibly share some insight with me as to why the loss of interest had occurred.

My friend said it was simple. He told me I had made it too easy for the guy and that I didn't require him to work to gain my affection. At first, I didn't really understand what my friend meant. Then he told me, it's as simple as this: you don't value anything that you don't have to work for. Obviously, I get it now, and I understand this concept applies to other areas in our lives.

The fact is, it applies in weight loss as well. Losing weight took a great deal of effort on my part. I successfully lost over ninety pounds six years ago and have consistently managed to keep it off. The hard work that I put in had a payoff. The payout was that I was successful in reaching my desired target weight. The success that I experienced caused me to be extremely pleased with and confident about my appearance. My energy level is high, and I feel just as good as I look. The end results were totally worth the effort it required.

Aside from all of the benefits that the weight loss brought me, I place a great value on the effort that I put forth. It has been the value placed on that effort that has continued to keep me on track in maintaining the results. You will work to get the results that you want, but it is important that you place significant value on the effort you put forth. We all place great value on things that we have to work for. You will be required to put forth much effort to lose weight, but the key is to remember this: I made it, and you will make it too!

CHAPTER 3

How Did I Get Here?

Knowing how you got to any place is important for two reasons. First, knowing how you arrived at a place will help you to understand how to move away from that place. Second, once you can identify how you got to that place you can then control the behavior that first led you there.

Obtaining wisdom and understanding are key components for any journey that you may find yourself on in life—not just weight loss. Knowing how you arrived at a particular place allows you to take responsibility for your role in getting there. You will need to own the responsibility that led you there.

During my childhood I developed some very unhealthy eating habits. As a child, I was not responsible—or at least I should not have been responsible—for setting boundaries for establishing healthy eating habits. In my opinion, healthy eating habits for children should be managed and established by their caregivers.

My parents divorced when I was a young child, so I was raised jointly by my grandmother and my mother. During that time, people were not as conscious of childhood obesity as they are now. There were many reasons for the lack of health consciousness back then, a key one being that children played outside far more than children do today—and playing meant exercise.

As best as I can recall, we almost always played outside. Yes, things were totally different in my childhood. Neither my friends nor I had an iPad, a cell phone for texting, an Xbox or Wii console for gaming, or any of the other technological gadgets that children have the pleasure of enjoying these days.

We simply had fun the good old-fashioned way, through vivid imagination and play. Most of the games that we played didn't involve anything more than an explorative mind, a lot of laughter, and an intense physical workout.

An all-time favorite game for my cousins and me was Mr. Freeze Tag, which consisted of one person standing on my grandmother's front porch while everyone else spread out in the front yard. The porch was considered home base; this meant you were considered "safe" if you actually made it there. I was generally picked to play the role of Mr. Freeze. This role was not by choice; it was assigned more so by default simply because I was the youngest. Initially, the game would start with Mr. Freeze (me) turning his (my) back on the other kids while counting to one hundred. The other kids would then scurry away to run and hide.

Mr. Freeze would leave home base to chase after and tag the other kids. If you could successfully make it to home base you were considered "safe." This meant that Mr. Freeze wasn't allowed to tag you—that is, freeze you. Otherwise, if you weren't quick enough and Mr. Freeze was able to tag you, you would then be frozen solid in your tracks.

Anyone who could successfully make it to home base was safe to hang out there until he or she could secure a clear path to tag and "unfreeze" those who had been tagged. The bottom line is that

Mr. Freeze was very busy, actively running around and chasing everyone.

Reflecting back on my childhood, I can't recall many children who were overweight. It was nearly impossible to be overweight back then, as there was so much physical activity engaged in during playtime. Yet, I managed to be one of the few that suffered from a weight problem. Playing the role of Mr. Freeze on a regular basis apparently wasn't enough to keep my weight under control.

The problem started when my single mother took a job on the second shift. Her schedule was 3:00 p.m.–11:00 p.m., making it impossible for her to provide parental care for me and my siblings during the evening hours. Instead, we were entrusted to the care of my grandmother, and we stayed with her each evening until my mother would return home from work.

Every day the routine was the same: my grandmother would cook dinner for us, then much later that night we would have dinner with my mother when she arrived home.

When I say "we," I actually mean "me"; my siblings would go to bed when we arrived home. I, on the other hand, would stay up and have dinner with my mother so I could spend time with her. It was my second meal for the evening. I can honestly say I wasn't hungry; I would eat simply because the food was there and because I was allowed to.

I am a single mom now, and I understand that when you are working to provide and care for yourself and your children some things may become less of a priority for you. I make that point to assure you that my mother was not intentionally neglecting her duty to regulate my food intake; she just simply didn't place a great deal of focus on how much I was eating. She was providing for a family, and I am sure she felt she had bigger fish to fry than counting my calories.

I have better understanding now as to how my mom may have been feeling. As a single mom, you may find yourself maneuvering through the impacts of divorce. You may be overwhelmed by the pressures from work. You may simply be flustered with the fear of being a single parent. There is an array of fears, issues, and problems that can prevent a single parent from making the best parenting decisions. I believe that an unbalanced mind always produces unbalanced decisions.

Don't get me wrong; it's not that my mother didn't want me to be healthy. The truth is, the potential impact of my poor eating behavior was actually not obvious to her. My mom had no idea of the implications that my second dinner had on my health. There were consequences to my eating patterns, but Mom was completely unaware of what they were.

As with any bad habit that you develop, there are likely to be consequences, and poor eating habits are no exception to this rule. Over time, as my pattern of eating dinner twice continued, I began to gain weight, and eventually I became overweight.

By the time I reached the age of nine years old I weighed over one hundred and sixty pounds. That's forty pounds shy of weighing two hundred pounds at the age of nine! I even acquired a nickname from my family. Because I ate multiple servings per day, my uncle began to refer to me as Pig, and soon thereafter other family members joined in. Before long no one in my family referred to me by my name anymore; they were all calling me Pig. Now, I can assure you the nickname was not intended to be reflective of my appearance. My uncle wasn't trying to be mean, but he actually thought I ate too much, and he voiced his concerns.

In case you are wondering—and just for the record—as horrible as it may sound that my family referred to me as Pig, I suffered no long-term damage to my self-esteem. It is currently intact and very healthy.

To put things into perspective, to show how much I ate as a child, I will share a very personal experience from dinner one evening. I can recall having dinner at my grandmother's and asking for a second serving. My aunt refused to serve me any additional food. My grandmother insisted that my aunt comply with my request, stating that I wouldn't ask if I weren't still hungry. This was actually farthest from the truth—I was greedy, not hungry. I can remember the look on my aunt's face, and can even hear her voice as she refused to accommodate the request.

Out of frustration, my aunt turned to my grandmother and said, "*No*, Mom, just look at her. I won't give her anymore food to eat, she's had enough!" My aunt was absolutely correct. I wasn't hungry; I simply had created a bad habit of having seconds, thirds, and sometimes fourths. This excessive consumption of food was hurting me and no one else, and someone clearly needed to do something about it.

I would like to tell you that my mother and my grandmother eventually sat down and discussed a plan of action to help me lose weight. Unfortunately, that never happened. Nor did they devise a healthier eating plan for me that eliminated my second dinners.

So what actually did happen? As with most activities in childhood, we eventually outgrow them, and that's what I did. By the time I reached the age of twelve, I began playing basketball in junior high school. I didn't get to spend much time on the court, but I did manage to get an extensive work-out every day at basketball practice. After a few runs of the "suicide" drill, I began to shed the weight.

In retrospect, playing basketball was one of the best decisions that I made in my youth. I didn't think so at the time, but it was; becoming physically active paid off in a big way. Later on I was fortunate enough to not struggle with being overweight again until my early thirties.

You will need to come to terms with where you are currently. Perhaps you arrived here by way of bad eating habits. These habits may have been an ongoing issue for you since childhood. You may be someone who is an emotional eater. You may be a compulsive eater who snacks while you are on the phone, only to catch yourself eating the last cookie as the call is concluding. You may even consider yourself to be addicted to the pleasure of sweets.

Or you may be someone who celebrates with food, or you may find comfort in food. Possibly you are the companion eater who allows food to fill in where human companionship is lacking. Then there is the person who is just plain old greedy. Ask yourself: Is that me? Do I simply eat it because I see it?

Maybe you are still struggling with the last ten, fifteen, twenty, or whatever number of pounds still hanging on after having children. Whatever the case may be, you will need to acknowledge it and own where you are right now.

Be honest with yourself and learn to face the root cause of how you actually got here. Speak the reasons out loud, even if there are multiple reasons; speaking your thoughts out loud gives life to them. This will make you more aware and conscious of your thoughts. After you speak your thoughts out loud, accept that you are here now. Release any feelings of guilt and shame; know that you will not remain at this place.

Going to a new place will require *growing* to a new place. Growth and change are synonymous, and change is constant. This means that along your journey you will be constantly changing and growing.

You may find yourself in one place today, but that does not mean you have to stay here. You have the ability to move to any place that you desire. If you see yourself moving from a size 20 to a size 8, know it's possible. In order to propel yourself forward you will need to know that yesterday ended last night and today is a new day. The power to create change is well within your reach today. All things are possible for those that believe.

There is power in taking personal ownership and responsibility for things that you have control over. I believe claiming ownership for where you are now is necessary in order for you to stretch, grow, and produce a more positive change in your future.

So, how do you take responsibility and ownership for where you currently are? Simply look in the mirror and repeat these two declarations out loud.

1) I *like* where I am, but I *love* where I am going.

2) I will embrace where I am until I get where I want to be.

Honestly, you may actually not feel as though you like where you are, but that's OK because moving to a new place is well within your reach. If you have any negative feelings about your current appearance, then release those thoughts. Begin to embrace where you are to improve your current feelings about how you look right now.

A positive attitude is pivotal in being successful at anything you set out to accomplish. If you begin the journey in a rut, it will take that much more energy to persevere and push your way through. By embracing yourself in the *now*, when you experience a setback along the way, you will be less likely to give up.

The acceptance of yourself in the now will encourage and motivate you to remain inspired to make positive consistent changes as you reach each goal. A positive attitude toward yourself will also allow you to let go of pressures that you may unknowingly place on yourself to achieve quick results.

If you are not ready to fully embrace where you are, you can change how you may be currently feeling by making the following confessions daily.

Confession #1: I arrived at this place by my own doing.

Confession #2: I take full responsibility for my current behaviors toward food.

Confession #3: I claim ownership and control of my life to make healthy lifestyle changes.

Confession #4: I am wonderfully and beautifully made in the eyes of God.

Confession #5: I am the only person responsible for my success.

Confession #6: Change is constant; it's from within; I cannot experience growth without change.

Confession #7: When it comes to believing in myself, I know that second opinions are not needed.

Confession #8: I will improve my self-image by presenting myself the way I desire others to see me.

Confession #9: I will be winning or learning on my journey, but never losing.

Your behavior will be driven by your current beliefs. The things that you believe about your appearance are derived from your past experiences and feelings.

As you improve your feelings about yourself, your beliefs will begin to shift and change. This will result in a more positive mindset, thereby improving your self-image.

Begin to visualize the new you and how you want to appear to yourself in the future. Seeing something visually in your mind will help to make the image more realistic. If you have an image that resembles the way you want the new you to look, then tape that image on your mirror.

Make it a point to look at the image daily and allow it to inspire you. Visual images will motivate you to keep pressing forward on your journey. It can be a picture that was taken at a time when you were happy with your appearance; a more personal image will help to boost your positive energy. But the image does not have to be one of you; a less personal image can also work as inspiration.

I can recall how I felt before I began my own journey. I would dress each day to go to work; my stomach would extend over the waistband of my slacks. Needless to say, this look made me feel less than pleased with my body. I had my fair share of love handles. At the time I didn't know how to embrace where I was. This made my journey that much more difficult. The truth is, all I knew is that I wanted to get rid of the current me and replace it with something more appealing.

I would go to a place in my mind where the handles didn't exist and I would visualize my body that way. It's been six years since I shed the ninety pounds and kissed the love handles good-bye. Visualizing how I wanted to see myself was a motivating factor in giving me the inspiration that I needed to get me started. Remember, it will require motivation, discipline, and commitment in order to reach your goals.

You will need to see it to believe it. Even if it doesn't feel like it now, you will succeed and reach your goals; you will obtain the results that you desire. Begin to ignite your motivation by visualizing where you want to be, and begin to move yourself forward in that direction.

CHAPTER 4

Start Small

When I think of the importance of starting small I can recall many times in my life when starting small didn't mean ending small. If you don't believe that starting small comes with benefits, you are in for a huge surprise. Many things that begin well tend to end well. Starting small actually increases your chances for success. If you are wondering how this is possible, then allow me to elaborate. One way in which starting small is beneficial is that it allows you to avoid taking on more than you can actually handle, thereby reducing your risk of failure.

Over a year ago, my doctor suggested that I needed to incorporate some type of physical activity into my daily lifestyle. As a working single mother, I didn't have any idea as to how I could rearrange my schedule to accommodate a fitness routine at a gym.

My doctor understood that my schedule was rather hectic, so he wanted me to choose an activity that I could easily maintain on a consistent basis. After all, how many times have you actually joined the gym only to find excuses later as to why you didn't have time to go? I am guilty as charged of doing this in the past—many times.

The doctor and I both agreed that a walk around the neighborhood would be a reasonable start for me. He just wanted me to get started doing something. We didn't set a goal as to how long or how far I would walk. His recommendation was that I simply just start walking and then go from there. For three weeks I thought about walking. I imagined myself walking; I could visually see it happening. Unfortunately, I never actually could motivate myself enough to actually do it. I simply just couldn't get started. I completely lacked the motivation that I needed.

Three weeks later I returned to the doctor for a follow-up visit. He inquired as to how the walking was going. I was embarrassed to tell him that I had not been able to get started, but at least I told the truth. The doctor didn't appear surprised at all; he seemed to have known the answer before I even confessed it.

The doctor asked me where I planned to walk. I told him that my plan was to walk around the lake in my community. He then asked me how long it would take me to walk to the lake and back. I told him possibly forty minutes, I really wasn't sure. After all, I hadn't actually done it yet, so I didn't know the answer.

He then told me the reason I wasn't walking was because I had subconsciously told myself the lake was too far away. He then suggested that I no longer consider walking to the lake. His recommendation was that I go no farther than the front door. Initially, I assumed he was joking, so I chuckled at his response. I soon realized he was actually serious. He simply wanted me to make it out the front door—period.

The doctor told me that in order to get started, I actually needed to start small, and the first small goal should be to simply make it out the front door. He said that as soon as I was successful in making it out the front door I should turn around and come right back in the house. I was to do so with the understanding that the goal for that day had been met.

He told me that he wanted me to try this for a few days; then he wanted to me walk to the stop sign at the end of the street. He told me that with each short goal that I accomplished I should strive to set a new one. My goal would be to go a little farther each time, but only when I was ready.

The first few days I put on my fitness gear and sneakers, and simply went out the front door. With each attempt, I turned around and came right back in. In my mind I was thinking it was too easy. It seemed far too simple, but the reality is I was actually doing it. I soon found myself going farther and farther, and it wasn't a problem for me to do so. At first it was to the stop sign, then the mailbox, then the next block, and after a few days I was able to increase the distance as well as my momentum.

After one year I was able to increase my walking time to an hour or more. I would walk even if it was raining, windy, and freezing cold outside. After one year my commitment to walking became solid. Walking became a habit. Once I created that habit and established it, I quickly realized that nothing could keep me from walking as a part of my daily routine.

Today I no longer walk in my community. I now look forward to actually going to the gym and running on the treadmill. Currently, I am averaging running over four miles per day, six days a week. The moral of the story is, I started small and increased my pace as I went along. I didn't just jump right in, thereby limiting my success. Starting big can make it more difficult for you to stay on track and focused. If you lose your balance, stumble, and fall, it may not be easy to pick yourself back up. Falling is generally easier than getting up. Starting small decreases your chances of falling in the first place.

Thinking back on the situation, I realize that it wasn't that I didn't want to walk—I actually did. I unfortunately lacked the motivation to get started. But by starting small I eliminated the pressure and anxiety that I was creating for myself internally. I believe that deep down inside I dreaded the thought of walking to the lake. Perhaps in my mind it did seem too far. Whatever the case, it was clear that I initially couldn't force myself to do it. I have now developed a consistent behavior that I actually enjoy and not one that I dread.

My ability to succeed in working out was ignited by my motivation to get started, but discipline and commitment have been the fuel that keeps me going.

I know when it comes to weight loss you may want to jump in full speed ahead. If you aren't convinced that starting small will yield good results, then I'll show you another way to think about it. Years ago, I purchased my first home at the age of twenty-four. After the purchase, I devised a "start small" decorating plan to furnish it.

It was my first home, and I wanted to make sure that I made the best decisions after the purchase. Shortly after I moved in, I had a vision for how each room should be decorated. My plan was to furnish the house without applying for any credit to do so.

I planned to put a large television in my upstairs game room. I envisioned a very elegant dining room that would contain nothing but off-white furniture. My bedroom would contain a large canopy bed. Unfortunately, when I moved in to my new home, I soon realized I had vision minus money. I had depleted all of my funds during the sale closing. I was completely tapped out.

Instead of making any of the purchases that I had planned, I decided to not purchase anything. I made no purchases for the first three years in the house. I didn't buy anything major. I didn't even splurge on blinds for my windows. Instead I used paper blinds from Home Depot. Yes, it's true; I had paper blinds for three years.

My thought process told me that if I didn't have the money for the furniture I would simply wait. I devised a plan in which I would make the furniture purchases each quarter with my quarterly bonus. This allowed me to purchase each item that I wanted to create the look that I had envisioned. I was able to make all the purchases without charging a single item.

The end result was that by starting small I didn't create any debt for myself. I was patient, and it took much sacrifice on my part. Starting small produced a desirable outcome in the end.

My reward for starting small was being able to have a lifestyle that was free from the stress of debt. I had to sacrifice to be able to do this, but sacrifice produces rewards. A little sacrifice goes a long way, but it requires that you must exercise a bit of patience and self-control.

I was able to apply this same philosophy to my weight-loss journey. I will discuss the rewards of sacrifice in greater detail in chapter 5.

Many of the people I spoke to during the writing of this book expressed to me they had placed much anxiety on themselves in a desire to achieve quick weight loss results. If you fit this category, shed the idea of quick weight loss, as well as the anxiety that goes along with it.

Quick weight loss sounds appealing, but it's not realistic for long-term goals. Making a lifelong commitment to healthier eating requires a mind-set change. I don't believe changing mind-sets can happen quickly, and I am sure that many of you will agree with me on that point.

You will need to adapt your mind-set to getting away from believing that you can change your eating habits overnight. I know it may take you some time to fully embrace this notion, but quick weight loss is not sustainable over the long run. Many celebrities' weight loss endorsements have fizzled quicker than the ink dries on the endorsement checks. Even with millions of dollars on the line, weight loss is a struggle. But I am here to tell you that it doesn't have to be.

Effectively changing your mind-set toward food requires you to apply deliberate, intentional, and consistent effort toward your behavior. Unfortunately, there is nothing quick or easy about making a change that will last a lifetime. It takes time, so have patience with yourself. Ask yourself if it is most beneficial to you to lose twenty pounds in four weeks and regain it in four months or to lose twenty pounds more slowly and keep it off for four years and counting.

Although work is required on your part, changing your mind-set towards food is not impossible. By taking deliberate actions I was able to begin a lifelong journey to eating healthier, and I have not looked back.

I encourage you to set realistic goals for yourself. Your objective is to start small and remove any goals from your plan that place too much pressure on you. Placing too much pressure on yourself will prevent you from feeling the motivation that you will need to begin moving forward. You can enhance your goal-setting as you progress, but remember to start small!

Keep in mind that the idea is to change your lifestyle and adopt a healthier way of eating. That means that any lifestyle change that you make should be able to be maintained permanently. You want to make changes that will last you longer than six to eight weeks or even six to eight months.

Ask yourself why you would rush a lifelong decision that could impact the rest of your life. It is best to take your time when making any decision that is intended to be permanent. By taking your time you increase your chances of getting it right, which means obtainable success.

You will need to be totally committed to yourself and to putting forth the effort to take intentional action. Otherwise you will find yourself attempting the journey over and over again. I don't want that for you, and I am sure you don't want it for yourself.

Think back in your mind; how many times you have started this journey, only to find yourself at the starting line once more? Tell yourself that you are one hundred percent committed to your journey, and mean it. Keep in mind that anything worth having is worth working for.

I want to further drive home the point about being patient with yourself. During the interview process, I asked one woman if she was putting pressure on herself to lose forty pounds, her weight-loss goal. She was very honest and told me yes. She said the pressure was actually causing her stress. I asked her to release the pressure by telling herself that she didn't have to lose the weight quickly.

I suggested that she pick a focus and stay there. I wanted her to understand that the actual results should not be her focus. The weight loss would be a benefit, but it should not be the focus. By removing the focus from the weight loss itself you can free yourself from feelings of stress and pressure to lose weight.

She told me that once she released the idea of doing things "quickly" she felt as though a burden had been lifted. When you desire to lose weight, focus on freeing as many negative hindering thoughts as you can from your mind. This will allow you to focus your energy on what's important, and that is making a sustainable lifestyle change.

Replay in your mind all of the diets that you have experimented with in your life. If you have never dieted multiple times, then good for you, but I can remember all the different times I have started the journey with no long-term success. I found this to be the case especially when my focus was centered on quick results.

I didn't obtain the desired level of success until I fully changed my mind-set and embraced making a lifestyle change as my focus. Don't get me wrong, the quick-results diets always produce short-term success. The problem is, I was never successful at sustaining consistent results for long periods of time. With no mind-set change, I would eventually resort back to bad eating habits and behaviors.

The consistency in my results only came when I made a conscious decision to change my relationship with food and how I behaved toward it. Once I changed the way I interacted with food, the consistency became a permanent part of my daily lifestyle.

Allow me to elaborate on this point a little more. I can remember once I tried the South Beach juice diet. For forty-eight hours, the only thing I was allowed to drink was juice—absolutely no food. It was torture, and during that forty-eight hours I was starving. I cannot begin to tell you how badly I wanted a big juicy rib eye steak, a baked potato with butter and sour cream, and all the fixings. At the conclusion of the forty-eight hours, I couldn't wait to get my hands on the steak, and so I did. I ate it, every single morsel. My gain was literally nothing—my success gain, that is. I am sure I gained something, but it wasn't the something that I was hoping for.

Quick weight loss sometimes offers techniques that may leave you feeling deprived. In return, you overcompensate to make up for the feeling of deprivation by overeating at the first chance you get.

The key is to remove the feelings of deprivation from the equation, and starting small will help. Practice being committed to eating healthier so that you are committing to putting unhealthy eating habits behind you. Allow the unhealthy habits to exist in your past, but don't carry them forward on your journey.

Ask yourself why you would want to continue to do the same thing over and over but expect different results. Let's be realistic: something has to change in your current behavior if you desire results. After all, losing weight is not magic.

If what you have been doing has not been working to get you where you want to be, then clearly it is time to try something different. I lost over ninety pounds, and have successfully kept it off for over six years. I can assure you that I did not do it by continuing to engage in the behaviors with food that originally caused my weight problem.

Because this chapter is focused on starting small I am not going to suggest that you drastically alter your eating habits. It would not be realistic nor would it be sensible for you to do that. Moreover, if you were to take that approach I suspect you may have the same reaction as I did regarding the South Beach juice diet. Drastic changes will leave you feeling deprived and falling off track quickly.

Depriving yourself is not the objective; changing how you view and interact with food is. You want to make sure that the changes are something that you can sustain without relapsing.

I will now share some easy and practical principles that I have been successful in maintaining. Portion control is very important in having a healthy relationship with food. It is also a key component in maintaining a healthy weight.

You will need to become aware of what a reasonable portion is, and then you will need to practice having control over your portions. Serving sizes exist on packages for a reason. It is there to allow you to know exactly what you are consuming with each serving. You will need to be deliberate in your portion control and serving sizes.

If you are having potato chips, take the time to look at the package to see how many chips are in a suggested single serving. Begin working toward managing your portions. Instead of reaching your hand into the bag, take the time to be aware of how many chips you are actually consuming. If it were not an important fact, the serving size would simply say one serving size is equal to one handful. I have yet to see a single serving size of one handful. With this being the case, be intentional about not just reaching into the bag and grabbing a handful.

Weight loss requires discipline, and part of that discipline is that you are aware of what you are eating and how much. I know the thought of counting calories may not be appealing to you, but as I mentioned earlier, a little sacrifice comes with rewards. Ask yourself what you are willing to sacrifice to obtain the results that you desire.

Here are a few suggestions that you can adopt at home as well as when dining out for making changes toward a healthier diet. These changes are small, but they will have a long-term impact on your success. They are simple changes, and should not be difficult to adopt; nor will they leave you feeling deprived.

Current Behavior	**Small Change toward a Healthier Diet**
Dressing on salad	Dressing on the side, dip into it
Fried foods	Prepare food grilled or broiled
Butter	Replace with olive oil
Soda	Replace with water
Sauces on food	Sauces on the side
Desserts	Fat-free or reduce fat desserts; or just say no

Coffee with creamer	Replace with green tea
Ice cream	Fat–free ice cream or yogurt, or with no sugar added
Juices	Replace with water
Red Meat	Replace with turkey/chicken/fish
Cheese	Light cheese made with 2% milk
Snacks	Healthy 100-calorie pack snacks
Baked potato	No sour cream or butter
Milk	2% or skimmed milk

These are minor compromises that I have made on my journey. You will need to make your own list of the top items that you are willing to compromise on. These items will be small sacrifices that come with a large reward. That reward is reaching the target that you have set for yourself.

As you identify items to substitute or alternate, the key is to start small. Set realistic goals that you can easily master; as you check the items off your list you will become comfortable with making additional changes. Later, as you master more and more changes, revisit your list to add new ones. If you add new items to your list weekly as you achieve each goal, you will realize that you are stronger than you thought you were.

Current Behavior   Small Change toward a Healthier Diet

CHAPTER 5

Sacrificing Your Way to Success

In chapter 4, I mentioned how advantageous the decision to start small was to me during the move in to my new home. If you look at that situation more closely, you can see that my willingness to sacrifice played a major role in my decision.

Starting small requires that you create a plan to ensure that you are able to reach your long-term goals. Looking more closely at my home decoration plan, it's clear to see the process I followed. To begin, I set goals for myself:

Goal #1: Avoid incurring debt to make purchases

Goal #2: Save money to purchase furniture

Goal #3: Purchase the furniture piece by piece

Goal #4: Decorate the rooms one by one

My goals were not complex; they were quite simple. The principles I used to furnish my home were also effective in setting goals to achieve weight loss. The key is that in order to move toward any goal, you will need to develop a plan of action to use as your guide. The plan of action that you choose will require that you apply deliberate action. You will not just fall into success. Success requires planning and follow-through. When constructing your action plan you will need to take into account all of the resources that can be used to aid you on your journey.

So how does planning help you to achieve your goals? Knowing what is needed to implement your plan of action is crucial to your success. Shortly after moving in to my new home, I began a job with an organization that offered a quarterly bonus structure. I decided that my plan of action for furnishing my home would require me to do so with my bonus pay. This would mean that I would have to wait until the bonus was paid out each quarter. The point is, I knew going in that my plan of action would require patience. To be successful on any journey, including weight loss, you will need to exercise patience and discipline to remain steady and on course toward achieving your goals.

If you remain steady and patient, you will then be able to check items off your action plan one by one. I mentioned that it took me three years to accomplish all of the goals toward completely furnishing my home. I could have taken a different approach and furnished my home much more quickly. I could have opted to apply for credit, and then charged all the things I needed. After all, I was fairly certain I would receive a bonus each quarter. I could have planned to pay the debt off as I received the bonuses. Have you ever done that? You may plan to pay something off when you receive some money, but then you find yourself needing to apply the money elsewhere when it arrives, negating the original plan. To be successful at anything, remember that it will require you to stay on your planned course.

If I had not remained on the allotted plan, I could have placed myself at risk of failing. There was the possibility that I could lose my job, resulting in the loss of my quarterly bonus pay. There were also a lot of what-ifs, but I decided to avoid these pitfalls, lessening my chances of being thrown completely off track. And if I had gotten off track, I would have accumulated debt, possibly falling in over my head.

The path that I took allowed me to reach all the goals that I set for myself. It also provided me the ability to hit targeted milestones that helped me to progress toward my goals. My plan of action required sacrifice. Simply put, sacrifice can be viewed as the will to give up one thing in exchange for something else. In reality, the thing that you are giving up has less value to you then the thing that you will ultimately gain.

While I talked with various people who are currently working to lose weight and eat healthy, the subject of sacrifice resurfaced numerous times. For many folks, sacrifice appeared to be a deterrent, something that was standing in the way of their obtaining success. Many of the interviewees shared with me that sometimes their unwillingness to sacrifice resulted in many setbacks along their journey.

To drive this point closer to home, I will illustrate how difficult it may be to sacrifice when you really don't want to. One night while having dinner with a girlfriend I experienced firsthand how challenging sacrifice is for some. After we completed dinner, my girlfriend suggested we ride over to Eddie V's Prime Seafood so that she could indulge herself in a blackberry cobbler.

My first thought was, why? My friend was attempting to lose weight. I wanted to keep her accountable to keep her on track. So I suggested that she skip the blackberry cobbler. After several minutes of debating back and forth, she simply stated she was going to Eddie V's Prime Seafood with or without me. The bottom line was that she was going to have the blackberry cobbler, and nothing that I had to say was going to stand in her way.

Stunned at her persistence to "cheat" on her plan, I went along with her to have her dessert. Clearly it was a losing battle for me. I sat quietly as she enjoyed the blackberry cobbler bite by bite. I was perplexed at her behavior, but I refrained from making any comments. The only statement I made was a silent one: I stood strong on my position to decline dessert.

I had already eaten dinner, I wasn't hungry at all. The benefit to having dessert was not that great to me, so I had made the choice to skip it; I had made a sacrifice. Sometimes you will be forced to ask yourself if the short-term gain is worth what you stand at risk of losing in the long run.

As I watched my girlfriend enjoy her blackberry cobbler, I began to realize that possibly her greatest roadblock was her inability to make sacrifices. My friend had identified clear goals that she planned to reach. She had also created a road map to follow to help her reach each milestone. Yet her unwillingness to sacrifice was pushing her goals farther out of reach. After three months, my friend lost only three pounds, and she was far from pleased with her progress.

My friend was clearly losing weight, but she was not losing at the rate that she had hoped for. You see, anything worth having is worth working for, and in many cases this means being conscious of sacrifices that you will need to make to achieve success.

Identify the goals that you would like to achieve on your journey. There is no right or wrong answer. Take your time, and be honest as well as realistic with your expectations. Your main goal may look something like this: I would like to lose twenty-five pounds. Being realistic in setting goals is important because it allows you to set targets that are within your reach.

The objective is to make changes in your eating habits that you can stick with. Give life to your goals by writing them down so that you can visually see what your goals are. I review my own goals in life daily, and I suggest that you do the same.

Lifestyle Changing Goals

Goal	Milestone	Target Deadline	Date Completed

Congratulations! Recognizing your goals is a very important part of the journey. Remember, goals are not action items. Identifying your goals will position you to create the best action items that will lead you to success in achieving the goals.

Now identify your weight loss milestones. You may need to revisit chapters in this book along the way for encouragement with the expectation that once you get started on the journey you will be able to stay focused. Practice reviewing your goals, milestones, and target deadlines as often as possible, preferably daily.

The milestones that you set at this time will help to measure your success as you move forward. This process of writing your goals, milestones, and deadlines down will also help to give you a sense of direction.

Think of your milestones as deadlines for your goals. Once you identify the milestone then assign a target date that you plan to complete the goal. For example, if you start your journey on March 14 and you have an ultimate goal to lose forty pounds, your first milestone may be to lose five pounds by May 15.

A second milestone may be to lose another five pounds by July 15. As these target deadlines are reached, mark each one as complete and move forward to the next goal.

You will need to be diligent and intentional in monitoring and keeping track of your progress. Based on the progress that you are measuring, you can then adjust your plan to better hit your targets. The more focus that you have on the journey, the more empowered you will find yourself; with this may come the feeling that you have total control of your results.

As you are measuring your success you will develop more and more confidence within yourself and in your ability to succeed. This journey does not end at a final destination. In keeping with that thinking, set your target weight as a goal, not viewing it as the end of your journey. Once you reach your target weight you will then need to work toward staying there.

You will celebrate successes along the way, but you cannot give up once your goals are achieved. Remember, this is a commitment for making a lifestyle change, and a lifestyle change will be long-term.

If you are unable to make changes that you can consistently sustain, you will find yourself starting the journey over and over again. Your success depends on taking deliberate action to achieve success, and in order to do this you must be willing to make sacrifices.

There will be some pitfalls along the way, and in chapter 9 we will cover workable solutions for overcoming pitfalls that may hinder your progress. Until we arrive at a point that you have sacrifice under control, let's focus a little more on your threshold for sacrifice. Soon, you will learn to effectively battle distractions that will ultimately hinder your progress.

Now ask yourself what is most valuable to you, and what you are willing to sacrifice on your weight loss journey. List the top areas where you will commit to making a sacrifice, and identify the benefit that the sacrifice will give you. This will help you to see the trade-off visually, giving the item you sacrifice less power and the benefit that you receive more power.

As you continue on the journey, your sacrifices will eventually no longer carry the same value as before. Initially, things that you list as sacrifices will seem like things that you are giving up. Over time, as you become more and more successful at changing your behavior with food, the sacrifices will fade and the benefits will remain.

Sacrifices   **Benefits**

CHAPTER 6

Discipline is in the Mind

In this chapter you will focus on understanding the importance of motivation and self-discipline. Believe me when I tell you that there is power in discipline, and it all starts in the mind.

Motivation and self-discipline go hand in hand. Motivation will allow you to lose the weight, but self-discipline will be your driving force in sustaining the results. These two traits are going to have a very significant impact on your progress.

I previously mentioned that I struggled with being overweight during two periods in my life. Aside from those two periods, I have also struggled with controlling and maintaining my weight for my entire life. I know all too well the struggle with that last ten pounds as well as the struggle with an extra ninety pounds or more. Those last few pounds might be considered less challenging to lose, but when you are working to shed the pounds, any amount of weight can be a struggle. The bottom line is that weight loss is just not an easy thing to do. The secret to weight loss is that there *is* no secret to weight loss. If you want to lose weight, it will require that you put in the work to do it.

Over the years, I have always been successful at shedding weight. It's the weight maintenance that I could never get quite right. It wasn't until I developed awareness as to how my inability to exercise self-discipline was hindering my success.

Self-discipline is simply exercising willpower over your personal desires. In this chapter I am going to work with you to develop techniques to enhance your ability to exercise self-discipline. These techniques will help you to successfully reach and maintain your goals.

Have you ever said to yourself, I just can't do it because I don't have any willpower? If your answer is yes, then you are not alone. I can remember over the years thinking those same thoughts, many times. There have been times in my life that I felt I lacked self-discipline, willpower, or self-control when it came to my eating habits.

Six years ago I became more aware of my thoughts and I learned to take control over them. This control allowed me to develop ways to change my behavior. Today, I am very much in control of my eating habits. The control that I have over my eating patterns is a direct correlation to my control over my thoughts.

Six years later, I no longer struggle with bad eating habits or weight gain. I have been able to successfully exercise self-discipline, and this has helped me to maintain a consistent healthy weight.

Looking back over the years, I can recall many failed attempts to turn my short-term goals into long-term results. When I moved from Raleigh, North Carolina, to Houston, Texas, I endured a major setback with my weight. During this time I was a size 10, and I was very comfortable with my size.

I adjusted to the move from small city to big city rather quickly. I was away from my family, doing new things and meeting new friends. I began to settle in to life in Houston very soon after my arrival. One adjustment that I was forced to make was going from a small variety of dining choices to an overwhelming number of selections.

At that time, in 1998, Raleigh lacked a variety of available dining establishments. However, upon my arrival in Houston, things changed for me. I was introduced to Tex-Mex, and it was delicious. I began to crave it, and I wanted it all the time—literally every single day.

Soon after meeting Tex-Mex, I was then introduced to southern Cajun cuisine. This flavor was new to my palette, and I simply could not get enough of it. In the words of Cajun chef and comedian Justin Wilson, it was delicious, I GUAR-RON-TEE!

Then I was introduced to a local favorite, Houston's restaurant. The Hawaiian rib eye was the best. I believe I dined at Houston's at least once a week.

Another favorite that I must mention is Tuesday nights at Birraporiettas. A group of my friends would join me there each week after work for the Fat Tuesday specials. But before long, as a result of my being introduced to new cuisines, old behaviors started catching up with me.

I soon realized I had a problem on my hands. Fat Tuesday began taking on a more personal meaning for me, and I didn't like the meaning at all.

I knew I had gained the weight, and it hadn't taken me long to do so. I could see it in all of my pictures. I was also aware that my clothes were no longer fitting. Many times I would try to squeeze into a size that was clearly too small. Within a matter of four months, I had gone from a size 10 to a size 14, and I was on the verge of needing to go up yet another size.

So what caused me to make a change? The turning point for me was a return visit to North Carolina for a Christmas holiday with my family. I was completely aware of my weight gain, but it really didn't hit home until I heard someone else acknowledge it. That someone else was my mother. As soon as she saw me, she gave me a swift pat on my rear and asked me, "What in the world have you been eating down there in Houston?"

The question echoed in my mind, as well as the answer, which I kept to myself: *everything*. I wanted to avoid the attention being paid to my weight gain, but it was impossible considering the entire family made it a focal point. It was continuously the topic of conversation. My childhood memories of being called Pig resurfaced with each mention of the weight gain. With bitter memories, I left North Carolina to return back to Houston feeling hurt, ashamed, and downright disgusted.

In reality, although I didn't welcome my weight gain receiving spotlight attention, it was still my truth. I had gained weight, and it was very noticeable.

In the introduction to this book, I shared a story about the reality check that Dr. Phil McGraw had given Oprah Winfrey and her girl-friends. The point Dr. Phil illustrated is that people are fat because they want to be fat. In retrospect, I can honestly say that Dr. Phil's theory was absolutely correct in my situation.

Dr. Phil's theory was applicable to me because I had gained weight and had no one to blame but myself. I didn't like the way I was feeling or looking, but I had chosen to do nothing about it. The only action that I took was to continue with the same behavior when I returned home to Houston. After my family acknowledged my weight gain, I was more aware of it than before, but I still continued the same behavior. I elected to not change a single thing about my eating patterns.

Reality didn't really hit me until one morning on my way in to the office. I stopped for breakfast at Jack in the Box as I did each morning. I had a daily routine to start each morning with a sausage/egg/cheese sandwich on a bun with hash browns and a Coke (non diet).

For some reason, this particular morning when I sat at my desk I felt embarrassed. I could actually hear my mother's voice echoing in my head, asking me what on earth was I eating in Houston. At that moment, I thought to myself, why are you eating this? Sadly enough, I had no answer. Although I ate it all, I didn't experience the usual satisfaction I had enjoyed every other morning.

Afterward, I looked down at my stomach and noticed the bulge over the top of my slacks. I thought to myself, this is the last time that I am going to eat at Jack in the Box, and it was. I don't recall getting much work done that day. I believe I spent the entire day asking myself how I got here. I honestly didn't have an answer, but I had arrived at this place, a place that I was not pleased with at all.

That afternoon I arrived home determined to make immediate changes in my eating behavior. My boyfriend at that time was an NFL athlete. Kevin was six foot three, weighed two hundred and forty pounds, and ate all the time. He would prepare dinner late at night after coming in from working out at the gym. I would enjoy spending time with him during a late-night dinner. These dinners didn't show on Kevin, but they were definitely visible on me.

That night I told Kevin that I was not comfortable with my body. He looked at me in utter disbelief, and his only response was, "So do something about it then." He said there was no sense in talking about it and that I needed to take action. Does this way of thinking sound similar to the point that Dr. Phil was making to Oprah and her friends? I do believe so.

Is it really that simple? If you don't like where you are then just do something about it? Apparently it *is* that simple because that's exactly what I did. That night I made a conscious decision to do something about it.

Kevin suggested that we go to the fitness center in the apartment complex after dinner. The next day we did it again, and the day after that and the day after that. We repeated our routine until it became a daily habit. The problem is, Kevin's workouts were intense. On some days I felt as though I were at an NFL training camp, and I didn't like it. I didn't like the intense workouts, and I didn't like Kevin's tough-love method of motivating me. I also didn't like being held accountable to go to the fitness center every day. It was becoming too much. I was ready to throw in the towel.

As time passed, I found myself watching my boyfriend walk out the door alone to work out. I missed a day here, then another, and before long I was no longer going at all. Inconsistent behavior will produce inconsistent results no matter what you are trying to accomplish in life. I lacked the discipline that was needed to remain committed to my goals. My motivation was gone as well, and I was unable to maintain any type of consistency with my workout routine.

Over time, due to some instances of ineffective communication and some unforeseen circumstances, Kevin and I decided to amicably part ways. I can assure you that the breakup had nothing to do with us not being in agreement on a workout routine. Afterward, I would sit in the apartment feeling alone and depressed about the end of my relationship.

A few weeks after the breakup I began to revisit the idea that I needed to lose weight. While sitting in the apartment alone one afternoon, I actually heard Kevin's voice in my head saying, "So do something about it then." I rose to my feet, and I spoke out loud, "OK, I will." As the words rolled from my tongue, my motivation was reignited once again, and this time the desire to win was much stronger than ever before.

Initially, I started working out on my own. I had been thoroughly trained on the things I needed to focus on in the gym. I followed the same techniques that Kevin had shown me, but now with far less intensity. First I started out working out early in the morning. After a few weeks, I added an additional afternoon workout to my schedule. Before long I was consistently working out both morning and evening, and the results were quickly evident.

I am not sure if it was my desire to look good so that I could enjoy an *Aha, look at me now!* moment, but I was definitely motivated. But it doesn't matter what the motivating factor is—for me or for you. What does matter is that if you don't like where you are, then do something about it! Don't just *think* about doing something, commit to yourself that you are going to willfully put action behind your thoughts.

If you do so, you will soon begin to see the results that you desire. And those results will begin to motivate you even more. My discipline began to increase, and yours will too as soon as you begin to see results—and I promise that you will. I was disciplined in the action that I took daily, and the payoff was worth it.

Today, make a conscious decision that you will no longer ignore, deny, or excuse the changes that you desire to make. Tell yourself the time has arrived to do something about it. You may or may not know what that something is, but if your roadblock is discipline, then don't worry, you will overcome it. I will help you.

I am committed to helping you to overcome your challenges with discipline. You will soon begin to experience results that will increase your ability to exercise increasing self-control over your eating habits.

The secret for people who are able to exercise self-discipline and self-control is that they actually believe in themselves. Allow me to illustrate this point for you. My friend Candis decided she wanted to shed thirty pounds. I was excited for her, and I offered to help her develop a meal plan. I offered to be her accountability partner, her motivator, and her encourager—in short, her personal support system.

Candis and I discussed her targeted start date, and she was soon on her way to success. Here is how Candis's journey began.

Day 1: She said she would start tomorrow.

Day 2: She said she needed to purge all of the "bad food" in her home and replace it with healthier alternatives. Again, she promised she would start tomorrow.

Day 3: She confessed that she worked late unexpectedly and had eaten badly at work, but she promised she would start tomorrow.

Day 4: She failed to respond to my text messages.

Week 2: She would not answer my phone calls or respond to any text messages.

Week 3: She would not respond to my e-mails, phone calls, or text messages.

I honestly wasn't trying to harass Candis; I was simply trying to do a good job at being her accountability partner. I was only checking in on her and her progress.

Candis's challenge wasn't that she didn't know what to do; we had mapped out a workable plan for her. Her challenge wasn't that she lacked motivation; she was fully aware of what she wanted to accomplish as well as the reasons why. She was indeed highly motivated.

Her biggest challenge was that although she knew what to do and why she wanted to do it, she didn't actually believe that she could do it. Her lack of belief in her abilities affected her thoughts. She thought she couldn't do it, and this thought led her to not even try. If you have any thoughts telling you that you can't successfully take the journey, free yourself from this way of thinking; let go of those types of thoughts. Negative thoughts serve no purpose other than to hinder your success, so release them.

A positive attitude, as well as your actions, must be focused and centered on believing that you can do this, and you can. I will be right here with you every single step of the way.

If Candis had only believed that she could really do it, then she would have allowed herself to get started. Instead, she was beginning the journey with feelings of defeat. I soon realized that she lacked the confidence that she needed to simply believe in herself. As you progress on your journey, you will see results, and the results will encourage you. As time progresses, your confidence will increase, and so will your self-control.

Keep in mind that discipline and self-control are learned, taught, and practiced behaviors; don't feel discouraged if you desire improvement in either of these areas. Both of these traits can be developed and enhanced over time. The change starts in your mind.

I know firsthand how difficult it may be for you to imagine being disciplined when it comes to food. If you enjoy a particular food, it may be extremely hard to imagine getting the taste of that food out of your mouth. Discipline is in the mind, not in the mouth.

One of my favorite foods is beef fajita nachos. If I am dining out, I order the cheese on the side, and I only consume a very small amount of it by dipping my nachos in it; I also request the dish without sour cream and guacamole. If I am at home I prepare the nachos with very little cheese. These may sound like minor adjustments, but the key thing to remember is that starting small produces big results over the long run.

A key component to practicing discipline is to learn to do something that you do not desire to do. The following challenges will help you to develop inner strength, and power over your thoughts. Over time the things that are most difficult to overcome will become least difficult. Focus practicing the following simple principles to discover your inner strength.

Think of it like this: All the minor small changes you make are like adding deposits to a bank. They may seem like small deposits, but over time they add up, eventually producing a big payoff.

Perform the challenges below, and as you master each challenge continue to select replacements so you can then incorporate new challenges into your daily lifestyle until you master all challenges. You will soon find that these things become ingrained within your normal diet routine.

Challenge #1: Select a dish you absolutely enjoy, then find or create an alternative version of it that is healthier.

> **Challenge key:** *To gain the most amount of power, it should be something you truly enjoy often, not something you are lukewarm about. A true sacrifice is giving up something that you really want, not giving up something you only kind of want!*

Dish _____

Alternative version _____

Challenge #2: Select a dish that you often enjoy, and choose an ingredient to eliminate from it.

> *Challenge key: To gain the most benefit, it should be something that is always a key part of that dish.*

Dish _____

Ingredient eliminated _____

Challenge #3: Select a dish that you often enjoy, and choose a healthier substitute for one of the ingredients.

> *Challenge key: To gain the most benefit, it should be something that is always a key part of that dish.*

Dish _____

Substitution made _____

Challenge #4: Select a dish that you often enjoy, and choose a healthier replacement.

> *Challenge key: To gain the most benefit, this should involve eliminating something that you have been enjoying for a long period of time.*

Dish _____

Healthy replacement _____

Now, create your own challenges and alternatives.

Challenge   **Alternative**

CHAPTER 7

No More Spinning Wheels

Have you ever felt yourself resembling a hamster running aimlessly in a wheel and getting nowhere when it comes to controlling your weight? I felt this way for many years, and I know firsthand that this feeling comes with a high level of stress as well as dissatisfaction.

Applying energy to run in a circle without seeing any movement forward toward some level of progress tends to cause feelings of helplessness in any situation, and weight loss is no exception. Experiencing feelings of despair and hopelessness may then lead you to abandon the journey altogether. When this occurs, the only emotion that is left is an overwhelming feeling of *why should I even bother?*

Spinning in a wheel is mentally and emotionally draining as well as exhausting. It leaves you feeling worn and tired. If you don't believe me, visualize yourself being in a career in which growth opportunities are nowhere in sight. If this resonates with you in anyway, then you will soon find yourself going to work every day feeling like a hamster in a wheel, running aimlessly but going nowhere.

To understand how spinning in a wheel will wear you down, let's take my marriage as an example. During my marriage, I felt as though I were putting forth great effort to make things work. While seeing no positive results or improvements in things changing, I began to feel completely drained. I was exhausted. I was far more tired than any hamster running in a wheel.

Spinning in a wheel can occur in any situation in which you are working hard and going nowhere. How many times have you started a weight loss plan, exerting lots of energy and effort, only to produce results that led you to feel drained, disappointed, or even hopeless?

It has happened to everyone, but it doesn't have to continue to happen to you. Today make a pledge to resolve to stop spinning in a wheel, and I will help you to do so. You will no longer exert energy and effort toward feeling that you are going nowhere fast. If you have been spinning in a wheel, you will now exit the wheel and begin to make steady progress.

Let's take a look at what the greatest causes of disappointment are along any journey. When expectation and reality are not aligned, disappointment is the gap that bridges the two together. Expectations come with a sense of hope. As the gap between expectations and reality increases, hope soon begins to diminish. As the gap expands, hope diminishes further, leaving behind a sense of hopelessness.

The opposite holds true when reality and expectations are more closely aligned. The gap between the two is lessened, resulting in a greater sense of satisfaction. One way to ensure success and satisfaction is to align your expectations closely with what is most realistic for you. Be as realistic as possible when setting your goals.

You may encounter periods when you will meet your expectations (i.e., what you are hoping for). At these times you will feel empowered and in control of your situation. The reverse of this also holds true: there will also be times when reality and expectations are too far apart. When this happens you may experience feelings of disappointment. When you are disappointed, you may also feel a sense of helplessness settling in, inevitably causing you to feel as though you want to give up. Readjust your expectations as needed, but never give up!

I'm not suggesting that you should lower your expectations or your goals. What I am suggesting is that you keep in mind this is a lifelong journey. Make an effort to select expectations that are more realistic, thereby increasing your chances for success.

One night while tossing and turning in bed, I decided to watch some late-night television. For the most part, the shows available in the middle of the night are infomercials advertising weight loss programs.

There have been numerous times that I have found myself scrambling from my bed in the middle of the night in search of my purse to order an ab roller, a dance beats video, a tummy tuck belt—well, you get the picture. My most recent temptation was during a Jillian Michaels infomercial, advertising her latest workout video.

I sat up in bed straight, feeling encouraged and motivated, and as soon as I heard a few of the successful testimonials, I was hooked. In my opinion, Jillian is a natural motivator. She can motivate anyone to do anything; I rushed out of the bed to search for my purse. I abruptly stopped myself in my tracks, and looked reality directly in the face. I set my purse down. I decided not to call that night to order Jillian's new video. Why? It wasn't realistic for me to do so.

Jillian has a great concept, and it works for many, but I had to be honest with myself. In reality, it wasn't going to work for me. No matter how bad I wanted to think that it could, realistically, I knew I wasn't going to do the work that was required.

So what do you do when you find yourself in this situation? The answer is quite simple. If you know deep down that something is not going to work for you, then find something else that does work. Take a firm stand against spinning in a wheel. Commit to goals that you believe are realistic for you. Not everything is for everyone; select goals that are realistic for *you* and stick to them.

In chapter 13, I will suggest an actual plan for you to follow. The plan will be your road map to success, but it will only work if you can follow the directions closely. I can't lead anyone who is not ready to go. If you are not ready to follow the plan, you will not be able to successfully stay on it. It's as simple as that.

The road map to success is going to rely on your ability to modify the road map to make it the most realistic for you. There are hundreds, possibly millions of diet plans available that you can choose to follow to lose weight. No one plan works for everyone. You will need to be careful in making selections that you believe you will actually follow.

One way to success is to select a plan to follow that has already proven successful for someone else. A plan that someone else has mastered can lead you down the road to success much quicker than following an unproven plan. So, how do you actually go about picking a good, proven plan?

It might seem easiest to pick the new, mainstream plan that everyone is talking about, but I suggest you refrain from doing so. Unless you are sure that plan is a realistic one for you, then you should avoid it.

I mentioned previously that at one point I attempted the South Beach juice diet. This diet lasted a total of forty-eight hours. I demolished a big steak at the end of that unsuccessful journey. Then there were the numerous times over the years that I tried diet pills that contained cascara sagrada bark.

At first, the pills appeared successful for the first few days as I could see immediate results. I soon realized the pills were causing me to lose water weight only. The initial results were apparent but also temporary. I shudder to think of the damage I may have caused to my body by taking the pills. They caused an irregular heart rate that would awaken me in the middle of the night, finding myself drenched in sweat and shaking. I can only imagine what possible liver, kidney, and heart damage I eventually would have experienced by continuing the usage of these pills over a long period of time. Let's just say they came with a few side effects.

Then there was the time my friend Amy went to her "fat" doctor and got a prescription for diuretics. She convinced me that we could eat whatever we wanted and the "magic" water pills would allow us to still be thin. This was another unsuccessful story, to say the least.

As I have stated previously, short-term quick fixes are never sustainable and will never produce the long-term results that you desire. Trust me on this one; I am speaking from a place of experience.

Using what has worked successfully for others is a faster, smarter, and more focused approach. Those who have already taken the journey and succeeded can offer a jump-start. Following in their footsteps can increase your level of success and leave you feeling that you are actually making progress. You will no longer feel as though you are staying in the same place, spinning in a wheel.

In 2007, on my first day at a new job I was carrying over two hundred pounds. I desperately wanted to shed the weight, but I didn't have a clue as to where to start. I was aware of all the plans available, but I didn't know which plan would prove to be the most realistic for me or would produce the results I wanted. The one thing I did know is that I was ready to make a change.

Every day I would observe my teammates' lunchtime behaviors. My team consisted of myself and four men. Three of them would stand near my desk at lunchtime and would discuss among themselves what they were going to eat.

I was intrigued by their consistency day in and day out. One day, out of curiosity, I inquired as to whether they were dieting or not. All three men told me that the prior year they had participated in a companywide Weight Watcher's challenge. After the challenge was completed, they each had been able to maintain successful results by continuing individual Weight Watcher's plans.

I inquired as to how much weight they each had lost; I was extremely interested in their success rates, considering that I desperately wanted to lose weight. One of the men told me he had lost forty-five pounds; another one had lost thirty pounds, and the third had lost one hundred pounds. My eyes glazed with excitement. I wanted to know more.

All three men looked great, and I couldn't believe they had lost that much weight in less than a year. I did what any unconvinced person would do, I asked for proof. You wouldn't believe it unless you had seen it with your own eyes. One of the guys pulled out a picture that was taken at his wedding. All three men were on the picture. The picture didn't lie; these men had shed the weight and they had kept it off with consistent, deliberate, and intentional behavior.

I now hope that you can better understand the reasoning as to why it's important to follow the plans of someone who has already successful taken the journey. It gives you the advantage of not spinning in a wheel. Think of it as preparing to run on a trail that you have never been on. As you begin on the trail you meet a person who just finished running on the same trail. This person stops and offers you insight as to where the potholes are, where to watch out for the stray dogs, and how to avoid the mud puddles. It is much more advisable to seek the wise counsel of those who have successfully traveled the path that is in front of you. Their wisdom can be a great benefit to you in your own travels.

One day I decided to speak to the teammate who seemed to have had the most consistent success in his journey. I wanted to get a better understanding of his eating behavior and patterns in order to incorporate them into my own plan. I was aware that consistency plays a major role in producing successful results.

I will discuss the actual road map in more detail in chapter 13. At this time turn your attention toward understanding how important it is to learn from the success of others. It will save you time, energy, and effort as well as improving your chances for a successful journey.

CHAPTER 8

Thinking it is Believing it

Over the last couple of years, I have learned from experience that my thoughts regarding food played a major role in my behavior toward it. Allow me to further explain. My interaction with food was influenced by what I believed about food. What I believed about food impacted what I thought about food. What I thought about food determined how I felt about food. And how I felt about food affected how I behaved with food. What does all of this mean? In a nutshell, it means that I had a very bad relationship with food, and it all stemmed from my beliefs, thoughts, and feelings about it.

Changing your mind-set regarding food will require that you change what you currently believe about food. Once you are able to change your thoughts and beliefs about food you can then change your relationship to it. Take a moment to ask yourself what you really think about food. Is it comfort, companionship, a friend? Answer the question honestly.

Recently, I stumbled across a very interesting article titled "African-American Women at Risk". Being an African American woman I wanted to read the article to understand what black women are at risk for. The article indicated that nearly 60 percent of black women were obese, compared with 32 percent of white women and 41 percent of Hispanic women.

I thought to myself that the title must be right based on the staggering numbers: African American women *are* at risk, and I had no idea before now. The article indicated that obesity had become an epidemic in the African American community, mainly among our women.

James Jackson, Director of the Institute for Social Research at the University of Michigan provided one possible reason as to why obesity in African American women was on the rise. He published his research in the *American Journal of Public Health*, citing that African American women often buffer themselves from chronic stress by eating "comfort food."

I totally can understand how food could be viewed as a coping mechanism to alleviate high levels of stress. Do you recall my friend Candis, who so desperately wanted to lose weight? Candis was excited; she was more than ready to get going. I could hear and feel her excitement. When the day came for her to start she was simply unable to.

I asked Candis if there was any reason for her delay in starting the plan that I had customized for her. She told me that she was stressed because her son had left to go and visit with her ex-husband for the holidays. She said that she felt depressed about her son's absence and she spent the night in the company of a pizza. She said she consumed most of it before going to bed to take her mind off how she was feeling. I am not sure if Candis was aware of her behavior, but it was clear to me that she was using food as comfort. We have all done it at one point or another. The objective now is to break the cycle; food can no longer be used as comfort.

Do you see how Candis's views toward food affected how she interacted with food? Based on her past experience, she had actually begun to believe that food was a source of comfort in her times of need. This led Candis to believe that food would actually make her feel better when she engaged in comfort eating.

Her thought pattern gave birth to her emotions regarding food. She felt that food made her feel better whenever she was feeling bad. Her desire for comfort resulted in her eating an entire pizza to ease the sadness that she felt when her son was absent from home.

Candis shared with me that this type of behavior with food always left her feeling much worse afterwards. This tells me that when food is used as a source of comfort, the relief is only temporary, and the lingering effects are far more damaging to one's emotional well-being in the long run.

I would imagine that African American women are not the only ones who find comfort in food when stressful times arise. Everyone suffers from some type of stress, regardless of race or gender. Be honest with yourself, and answer this question out loud: do you ever find yourself seeking comfort from food to ease pain, stress, or negative emotions?

If so, join the club. I have done it myself, many times in the past. As I have stated before, I am your friend and I am on this journey with you. There is no reason to feel any sense of shamefulness for doing something that is human nature and that others have done.

It is totally natural for any human being to seek the comfort of something when life becomes stressful. Some people choose shopping for comfort. Some people seek out support from friends. And some people seek comfort in food.

Whatever the case may be, if you have developed damaging beliefs about food that are affecting your current behavior, then please know that those beliefs can be changed. It will take work, but once you change what you believe about food, you can then change your relationship to it. Creating a healthier relationship will help to steer you in the direction of creating a more positive lifestyle change.

Take a moment to list what you believe and how you feel about food under various situations to determine the behavior pattern that you have developed toward food.

Exercise #1: When I feel sad

Belief	Thought	Feelings	Need to Fulfill	Behavior Change

Exercise #2: When I feel stressed

Belief	Thought	Feelings	Need to Fulfill	Behavior Change

Exercise #3: When I have personal relationship dilemmas

Belief   **Thought**   **Feelings**   **Need to Fulfill**   **Behavior Change**

Exercise #4: When I feel disappointed

Belief   **Thought**   **Feelings**   **Need to Fulfill**   **Behavior Change**

Exercise #5: When I feel excited

Belief   **Thought**   **Feelings**   **Need to Fulfill**   **Behavior Change**

Exercise #6: When I feel frustrated

Belief	Thought	Feelings	Need to Fulfill	Behavior Change

Stress is not the only emotion that will cause someone to seek comfort food. During the writing of this book, one of the people I interviewed shared with me that she had been an "emotional eater" all of her life, in good and bad times.

When I interviewed Stella, she told me that for the past thirty-plus years she had established a codependent relationship with food, and when she needed comfort she knew exactly where to find it.

She told me that her relationship with food was the same whether her emotional state was in a good place or a bad one. She would seek out comfort during both variances of emotions. I delved a little deeper into the meaning of emotional eating and how it pertained to Stella's personal journey.

Generally when you hear the term *emotional* used to describe someone's behavior, you tend to think of the person as someone who may be sad, crying, yelling, unsettled or all of the above.

Stella told me that this was not entirely the case with her. She said that when she had a great day as a result of good news, she would come home excited and seek out food to share her happy moment with. Then there were the low days, when things didn't go quite as planned. She would come home on those days and seek comfort in her food to divert the sadness she felt from being alone.

I asked her if she could articulate to me the feelings that she experienced whenever she engaged in "emotional eating." She took a moment to visualize the feelings, and then she said that whenever she was eating for comfort, she actually felt as though a pair of arms were wrapped around her, comforting her.

I asked Stella to explain to me how she felt after the comfort had passed. She told me that she was always left with a feeling of shamefulness and disgrace, thinking, why on earth did I just eat that? She said she was always conscious of her behavior while she was engaging in emotional eating, but she chose to do it anyway.

As we talked more I began to probe her for a deeper meaning as to what was really causing her to seek comfort in food. She eventually told me if she had a loving fulfilling relationship she would not feel the need to find comfort in food. She was actually fulfilling a need, an emotional need that she had for companionship. Now, the solution to Stella's problem is not an easy one. Unfortunately, finding a companion will not be as easy as snapping a finger. What she can do, though, is identify the emotions that cause her to interact with food in such an unhealthy manner. Then she can be proactive in her actions so as to not fall into some of the same traps she has in the past when encountering those same emotions.

Since Stella now knows that her need for comfort food is related to her desire for companionship, she can be proactive in her future actions. I advised her to seek support from friends during her good as well as her bad days. Today, if she were driving home and got a flat tire, I would imagine she would come in and eat a pint of ice cream to comfort her stressed nerves.

Stella may think that the temporary soothing feelings will lessen her frustration about the flat tire. By being more proactive in the future, when a stressful situation is encountered she can find better ways to handle it. She can choose instead to make arrangements to spend time with a friend to vent her frustrations.

Perhaps a friend will not meet the need of the desire for male companionship, but it will allow her to go home alone and not seek attention from food. This level of awareness will help Stella avoid a trap. Initially, this may not be an easy transition for her to make. It will take effort on her part, but the change is realistic and can be successfully undertaken.

Think about each behavior that you listed for the previous exercises, and then ask yourself what you are really feeding. What need are you really trying to satisfy?

Ask yourself if you are attempting to replace sadness, stress, disappointment, excitement, frustration or some other emotion (you can fill in the blank here). Once you have identified the need, write it down. Then identify an alternative that you can successfully use to replace your current behavior with another behavior, and write the behavior change down.

Changing how you behave with food will have a huge impact on empowering you to transform your current beliefs, thoughts, and feelings toward food. This will give you control to permanently change your interaction with food.

You have just reached a major milestone on your journey! You are now well on your way by having identified root causes for negative behaviors with food as well as alternatives for proactively offsetting those behaviors. Congratulations, you are definitely on the path to success! Now keep moving forward!

CHAPTER 9

Conquering the Pitfalls

Please allow me to share a painful personal truth with you. Six years ago, when I began my journey, the start was bumpy and far from anything I would consider graceful. My challenge was in actually making the commitment to get started. No matter how hard I tried, I just couldn't start.

How many times have you thought about starting a weight loss journey but were unsuccessful in the initial launch of it? Perhaps you mapped out a plan to lose weight in your mind but were unable to get that plan off the ground. You may have even been committed to your vision enough to go as far as enlisting others in your plan to offer support to you, yet still your progress was minimal. No matter how hard you tried, you were unable to ignite your motivation.

It happens, and it happens to the best of us. The reality is, once you make a commitment, you then have to put action to that commitment. Although hope carries with it much power, without action hope simply dwindles into a desire that never actually manifest into anything productive.

Take, for example, this book that you are reading. You may be holding it in your hand, reading it online, or perhaps on an e-reader, but whatever the case may be, you are actually reading a book that

I have written. The point that I am stressing is that I actually had to write this book before your eyes could glimpse the words on these pages. I have dreamed of writing a book all my life. I started a book in 2003, and after several months, I had completed part of it, but I never finished or published it.

As a matter of fact, the pages are still bound together in my bottom nightstand drawer. As the years passed I began to realize that time was going to continue ticking away whether I wrote the book or not. It became obvious to me that any delays in my progress were well within my control. I could have possibly spent the next three, five, or seven years hoping to write this book.

The book did not take on a life until I put action behind my commitment to actually sit down and write it. It was as simple as that. Anything that you are hoping to accomplish will require commitment along with action in order for you to achieve success. My point is that you can't just hope for something to happen, you actually have work to make it happen, and weight loss is no exception.

Today, make a promise to yourself that as you start your journey you will be committed to do the work that is needed to reach your weight loss goals. I mentioned that the start of my own journey was not an easy one. Don't worry about how long it will take you to achieve success at weight loss; place your focus on just getting started on the journey.

Although my start was rocky, I didn't allow myself to quit. When I first began, I often experienced disappointment, but I stayed on course. When I found myself knocked down along the way, I would simply get up and not give up. If I told you that staying on course was easy, I would be lying to you. The important thing to remember is that you are in this for the long run; stay on the path, stand strong, and you will succeed in reaching your weight loss goals.

So how do you overcome obstacles and discouraging moments when you find yourself face-to-face with them? I will tell you what worked for me to overcome obstacles, and it can work for you too. One weight loss obstacle that I faced was my showdown with a strawberry ice cream cake. My husband came home one afternoon with the cake, with no warning to me. I didn't have the willpower to resist my temptation to eat it. Don't get me wrong: I was committed and willing to do the work, but I was still faced with an occasional challenge. Commitment—even alongside with genuine effort—still does not guarantee you success along the journey. You will need to remain deliberate in your actions on a daily basis.

Even when you are working your hardest to stay on track, you will still be faced with pitfalls. Don't get discouraged when this happens; a pitfall is nothing major; it's simply a trap. When you are aware that a trap exists, then you can avoid falling into it by being more careful. You can, and you will, get around it. As long as you have the pitfall on your radar, you are in control.

In my situation, the strawberry ice cream cake was an obstacle, it was indeed a pitfall. I wasn't equipped to handle it when I was forced to face it. I sadly fell right into the trap. I gave in to my desire to eat the ice cream cake and, unfortunately for me, I ate the whole thing. I know what you are thinking, but stop! Remember, no judging is allowed! My point is that just because you encounter a trap doesn't mean you are doomed to fall into it. When faced with a trap, begin to practice the following steps: awareness, acknowledgment, and avoidance. You will soon have no trouble avoiding any trap you may come across on your journey.

So how do you guarantee that you will be able to stand firm on the path without being knocked off course by pitfalls? You can find the answer in a travel adventure that I experienced last year.

A friend of mine decided she wanted to celebrate her birthday at South Beach in Miami. We made hotel reservations, rented a car, and headed to Miami looking forward to a few fun days on the beach. Our hotel was a few blocks away from the beach, so each day we would drive a few blocks to hang out on the beach.

On the first day we headed toward Ocean Boulevard on South Beach. My friend was carefully following the instructions from the GPS system. Suddenly she was distracted by a detour sign on the street, and quickly made a right turn. The sudden turn took us off our planned course to the beach.

Neither my friend nor I were aware that we were off course until we heard the GPS system "rerouting." My friend quickly made a U-turn to get us back on track so that we could resume the planned course.

On the second day, we headed out to the beach again. This time, following the same GPS directions as before, for some reason—at the exact same location as the day before—we made the same wrong turn. We both were puzzled when the GPS system once again announced that it was rerouting.

We quickly realized the detour sign had thrown us off course once again. This time we didn't drive as far as the day before. We decided to make a U-turn much sooner.

On the third day, you wouldn't believe it, but at the same exact location as the previous two days, my friend made the same wrong turn. When we heard the GPS system rerouting, we both began to laugh. Without hesitation my friend quickly made the familiar U-turn and, once again, we resumed the course we had initially planned to follow.

On the fourth day, we were heading on the same course to the beach once again. Although we were traveling the same path for the fourth day we were still unfamiliar with the area, so we continued to rely on the GPS for guidance.

As my friend approached the detour sign that now had become very familiar to us, she said, "I refuse to make the same wrong turn again today!" This time she was aware of the sign, and acknowledged it before she approached it. She took deliberate action to avoid making a wrong turn. She was now more in control of making sure we stayed on the right course.

The lesson to be learned here is simple. By taking the same wrong right turn three days in a row we became aware of where the turn existed, allowing us to completely avoid it. If you know a wrong turn lies ahead, wouldn't you agree that the most logical choice is to acknowledge the wrong turn and go around it? You can choose an alternative route if you like, but the key is to take intentional action that will prevent from veering off your designated course.

In my travel experience, the pitfall was the detour sign that led us to repeatedly make the same wrong turn. Although we were able to quickly get back on track, we found it to be extremely frustrating to make the same wrong turn over and over again. Who wouldn't feel this way? Continuing to repeat the same unfavorable behavior is enough to frustrate anyone.

How many times have you started your journey to lose weight and keep it off only to find yourself getting thrown off course by a pitfall? You may very well know where the pitfalls are, but you fall into them just the same. Remember, falling into a pitfall is completely normal. Practice putting your focus on avoiding all traps that you are aware of on your path.

You will need to identify known pitfalls that you may encounter along your journey. Find an alternate solution to avoid the pitfall; this will save you time, energy, and frustration and will help to keep you focused and on the right path.

Avoiding pitfalls will allow you to progress to your desired destination much faster and with more ease. You will need to be aware of the pitfalls to not repeat the same actions that force you to fall. If you find you have fallen, be patient with yourself as you climb out. Get up and get out of the trap, but never give up on yourself.

During my journey, I have fallen into pitfalls many times. When I did so, I didn't stay on the wrong course for long, nor did I allow myself to make an excuse to get off course. I simply picked myself up and remained steadfast on the journey.

I didn't give up when I found myself making a wrong turn, and you won't give up either. If you find yourself faced with a pitfall, it's OK, you will get back on track and keep moving forward until you can avoid such pitfalls altogether. It may take a little time or it may take a long time, depending on how big the pitfall is for you. But once you are aware of a trap, it's no longer a trap. You have control over the trap by being aware of it, allowing you to avoid it.

If I had known my husband was bringing an ice cream cake home, I could have politely asked him not to do so. I could have explained to him that my self-control was not established enough to resist indulging in my desires for the ice cream cake.

It's always easier to say yes to things we desire than it is to say no. Keep in mind that pitfalls are temporary challenges on the journey and not permanent roadblocks. This means a pitfall is not the end, nor does it have the power to end your success. Pitfalls are detours, and yes, they may slow you down, but please don't allow them to halt your progress. When faced with a pitfall, resolve to get on track and to stay there!

It is also important to refrain from getting discouraged by pitfalls. As you overcome pitfalls you will learn to be more patient with yourself and your perseverance will increase, allowing you to come out victorious in the end!

Here are a few pitfalls for you to look out for on your journey. These may resurface along the way, but as long as you are fully aware you will be able to face them head-on, empowering yourself to avoid them altogether. Gaining control over these pitfalls will strengthen your ability to overcome other pitfalls along the way, thus increasing your chances for success that much more!

Pitfall #1: Travel

Prior to traveling, research restaurants where you plan to dine, by doing so you will be able to make healthier selections. Blindly searching for dining selections may force you to select places that are way off course (i.e., detours).

Prior to traveling to West Palm Beach a few months ago, I decided to dine at Seasons 52. The food was delicious, and nothing on the menu was over four hundred and fifty calories. Being equipped for the journey simply means being prepared. Equip yourself with knowing what you plan to eat ahead of time when dining out. If you are unprepared you may chose badly, taking yourself off course. Make sure you research ahead of time if possible.

Pitfall #2: The Influence of Friends

Now, this one may be a tough one. Please do not allow friends with bad eating habits to influence your behavior. It's easy to sometimes join in with the others and to tell yourself that it's OK to do what others are doing.

As the old adage goes, "When in Rome, do as the Romans." My advice is to *not* behave as the Romans behave when in Rome if the Romans are behaving badly! It may feel OK as you are engaging in the bad behavior, but trust me, when you knowingly veer off course, regret shall soon follow.

I once attended a Bible study event at a friend's home. At the conclusion of the Bible study she served us a full dinner that she had prepared. The menu was extensive: there was salad, seafood gumbo with rice, chicken cacciatore, and a selection of several side dishes and desserts. Everyone was more than happy to partake in the feast.

Some of the guest loaded their plates with seconds. Knowing that I was on a journey, I decided to ration my servings. I only selected what I considered to be sensible and within reason for me. My friend was offended that I didn't splurge and have a taste of everything that was laid out before me.

I explained to my friend that I don't just eat food because it is available. Sometimes you will find it is harder to say no to people than it is to say no to food. If you find this to be the case, then I don't want you to get discouraged and give into the "when in Rome" theory. Stand your ground as graciously as you can, because *you* are the only one who is responsible for your results—no one else. I am not sure that my friend appreciated my self-control, but she respected my wishes and backed off.

Pitfall #3: Dining Out

If you are not careful, this can be a major pitfall. If possible, before dining out, look up the menu online and download it. As with pitfall #1, you want to be prepared to make wise choices. Personally, when dining out I skim the menu for healthy selections as well as for adjustments that I may need to make to an entrée such as no cheese, no sauces, broccoli instead of rice, and so on. There are lots of hidden calories in the accompanying sauces. My general rule of thumb is to request all sauces on the side. If it's a sauce that you can do without, then save yourself the calories and skip it altogether. Otherwise, you can dip food in the sauce to sample it, but please do not eat the entire serving. The key is to be as prepared as possible before arriving at your destination when dining out.

Pitfall #4: Holidays/Special Occasions

I know that holidays and special occasions are almost always viewed as a "get out of jail free" card. The journey does not cease because Valentine's Day, your birthday, Christmas, or the Super Bowl rolled around on the calendar. Remember that consistent behavior will produce consistent results and the same holds true for inconsistent behavior. Stay focused and consistent along your journey. Please do not allow yourself to fall into a trap simply because of the day on the calendar.

Pitfall #5: Skipping Meals

Many people have busy schedules, and sometimes the planning and coordinating of dinner can be a challenge. Regardless of whether you are working in the home or out of the home, I am sure you have tons of other responsibilities to attend to on a daily basis; planning dinner is just one of them. If you factor in a family, with a significant other, children, pets, homework, extracurricular activities, and the like, the time in the day seems to diminish quickly. Make time to prepare your meals a top priority!

I know firsthand how a pitfall can deter you from the journey. Working in Corporate America and being the single mom of a very active six-year-old certainly makes my schedule very busy. I have juggled afternoon ice skating lessons, evening swimming lessons, cheerleading after school, and homework. Having many activities to attend can sometimes cause dinner to take a backseat.

The easiest thing to do sometimes is to pick up something fast, quick, and easy. This pitfall is one that many busy individuals are faced with. Do you recall Judith, the young lady who would eat badly if faced with any type of change? She revealed to me that when she was busiest she actually would forget to eat anything at all. Since she owns her own business, you would imagine that she would have a schedule flexible enough to take time for lunch.

Quite the opposite. On most days she missed breakfast, worked through lunch, and would eat junk food throughout the day to generate energy from a sugar rush. Many nights she would skip dinner completely because her appetite would be ruined from all the afternoon snacking on junk food. The end result was that she gained forty pounds over the course of two years.

My suggestion to Judith was to set a reminder on her calendar to eat breakfast, snacks, lunch, and dinner. Many times she worked late hours and was still in the office long after dinnertime. By setting the reminders and actually eating the meal at the appropriate time, she was able to proactively avoid the skipped meals pitfall. And as you now know, being able to avoid pitfalls will help to ensure that Judith can better stay on course toward reaching her desired goals.

How many times have you found yourself skipping meals? My general rule of thumb is to have a sensible breakfast, and then a healthy morning snack, which prevents me from overindulging at lunch. I always try to select a sensible, healthy selection for lunch. I also select a healthy afternoon snack, which prevents me from overindulging at dinner. It has been most beneficial for me to schedule the meals and snacks approximately two to three hours apart. This prevents me from feeling hungry throughout the day and being tempted by pitfall #6.

Pitfall #6: Sweets

After conducting several interviews I was convinced that, for some, sweets can be the proverbial "monkey on your back." I realized that a few people I interviewed actually have an uncontrollable obsession with sweets; in some cases the word *addiction* was used. For others, sweets felt like a burden.

Today avoiding junk food and desserts is very easy for me to do, but there was a time when avoiding sweets was not such an easy task. Remember my encounter with the strawberry ice cream cake? I can remember sitting in my bedroom being attracted to what seemed to be a voice calling to me from the kitchen. I would walk into the kitchen several times to look at the ice cream cake in the refrigerator. Each time the voice called to me, I would allow myself to indulge and take a small taste.

First it was just a taste from the corner of the edge of the cake. Then it was a sliver from the center and an occasional finger swipe. But eventually, after all the small taste-testing, the cake would vanish, leaving behind nothing more than resentment and disappointment.

I know that I am not the only person who has experienced the come-hither call from the kitchen by something sweet to eat. It may have been the Oreo cookies in the pantry that called you. It could have been the chocolate cake on the counter. Possibly it was the ice cream in the freezer. The scenario is generally the same in all situations. You hear the call, you go, you admiringly gaze at what you imagine will taste so good to you, and then you take a bite.

At that very moment your heartbeat slows down, you inhale, you exhale, and then you smile and think, this is so good. For one instant, you actually do feel good. Perhaps you may even feel a sense of relief. Then within a matter of moments you do one of two things.

You continue to eat more and more and more, and repeat the process until the entire sweet treat is completely gone. Or, your smile turns downward into a frown, and you begin to cringe internally, thinking to yourself, why did I just eat that? Your good feeling then soon leaves you, turning into a not-so-good feeling.

So how do you avoid the come-hither call? The answer lies in being proactive. If you know you will hear the voice calling you, then be prepared for it. Now, honestly, it's not an audible voice, but it's actually a thought that comes into your mind and it is strong. It may be so strong that it dominates all other thoughts. You can't seem to shake the thought and you definitely cannot ignore it. The more you resist, the more it calls to you, to your mind—until eventually you respond.

The emotions tied to sweets are very strong for some people. When the craving comes on it is sometimes impossible to ignore. If you are one of those individuals who craves sweets, the solution is to practice satisfying the craving, to fulfill it but not give in to it. What I mean is, *taste* the sweet, but don't *eat* it. By giving in to tasting the sweet you are eliminating the feelings of deprivation.

Many of the folks I interviewed shared with me that once they fulfilled the craving their needs were actually met. I am not going to suggest to you to quit sweets cold turkey, but please recognize that sweets are a pitfall. Instead of avoiding sweets altogether try to avoid the ones that you can't resist by finding a healthy alternative.

If this pitfall applies to you, then know that the monkey on your back will eventually climb off. It will simply require that you learn techniques to outsmart the monkey. Focus your attention on staying in your own lane when it comes to sweets. Practice tasting sweets that you can't avoid altogether to satisfy the craving, but do not fully indulge yourself by completely giving in to the monkey. Some things are meant to be tasted but not eaten.

Remember that you will be required to make choices and decisions along the journey, and they will result in consequences. When confronted with a tough decision, ask yourself if the piece of blackberry cobbler or apple pie, or the chocolate bar, or whatever the sweet is, is worth compromising your results. More than likely, your answer will be a resounding no.

Prepare to grab the reins and maneuver this particular road carefully and steadily; it will be a bumpy part of the journey, but you will not get knocked off course. Remember, discipline is in the mind!

Pitfall #7: Avoiding the Scale

I cannot express to you the number of times I have heard someone tell me how much they dislike the scale. In my opinion, the scale is the most truthful companion you will ever encounter. Your scale will tell you the truth regardless of what feelings are at stake.

Why do people avoid the scale? Many don't want to face the truth. Ask yourself how can you make a change for the better if you don't face your current truth, whatever that truth may be.

While interviewing Judith, I asked her if she weighed herself during the two-year period in which she gained the forty pounds. She said she refused to get on the scale. I asked her when she had noticed her weight gain. She said it became obvious to her in pictures that had been taken during that period.

I thought it were interesting that she could see the weight increase happening gradually but didn't do anything about it until forty pounds later. She told me that she didn't know it had reached forty pounds until her doctor told her so. I asked her if by getting on the scale it would have been easier to catch five pounds as opposed to thirty-five pounds, and her answer was yes. Since she had an aversion to the scale, she didn't know how much weight she was gaining.

If controlling your weight is a goal that you are setting for yourself, ask yourself how you can gain control over something that you're afraid to take control of. You may not like what you are seeing on the scale, but in order to take control over it you will have to face it. Stepping on the scale empowers you to take control of your weight. You may not like it, but it is your truth and you must own it in order to do something about it.

CHAPTER 10

You are Accountable

In chapter 3, you identified the eating behavior that led you to the place where you currently are. The objective was to acknowledge how you arrived here but not to allow yourself to dwell on those thoughts. Your purpose in knowing how you got here is simply to avoid those behaviors in the future. You can't correct bad behavior if you haven't acknowledged what the bad behavior is.

To better understand this concept, let's take a look at Judith's behavior. By acknowledging that any type of changes will send her off course, going forward she can be more aware of what to do when changes in her life arise. Her awareness concerning these changes equips her for success by avoiding certain behaviors before actually engaging in them.

The main point I want to stress to you at this time is that how you arrived here is only important for planning purposes toward obtaining successful results in the future. Acknowledge the behavior that has led you to this place and then move forward. By doing this you will move forward with more awareness. It is important to acknowledge the behaviors that hinder your progress; otherwise you will continue to repeat them. These behaviors are roadblocks that lie in your path of your road to weight loss success. You must hold yourself accountable in not repeating any bad behaviors that you currently engage in with food. You will be the only person responsible for changing your eating behavior in the future; it's as simple as that. Commit to being accountable to yourself by telling yourself that the only person who is in control of producing the desired results is you. Commit to being one hundred percent accountable to yourself.

I know many people who have taken the journey and experienced much success with the aid of an accountability partner. I recommend that you enlist the help of a friend, relative, spouse, or anyone else you trust to support and encourage you along the way.

Keep in mind your accountability partner's role is for support and encouragement only. This is *your* journey; you own it. Your accountability partner is not responsible for your results. I want to emphasize the accountability rules clearly because there have been many times that friends asked me, "Why did you let me eat that?" I would respond to the question with utter disbelief and silence.

It may be easier to project blame unto others who may be standing nearby when we fall short on the journey. If you want to be successful, then please do not fall into the trap of blaming others for your eating behaviors. Transferring misplaced blame to others is a pitfall; avoid it at all cost.

When my husband brought the strawberry ice cream cake home, I was quick to blame him after I ate the entire cake. I can even recall being angry at him. But he wasn't the one who ate the cake—I was. It was much easier for me to blame him than to allow myself to be accountable for my inability to exercise self-control. Again, I want to reiterate that it is much easier to say yes to something that you want than it is to say no.

I can recall one afternoon sitting around the kitchen table with a neighbor as she and I shared details of weight loss struggles. I shared with her that when I first started my journey, my husband would bring a package of Oreo cookies home several times a week. She looked at me and said, "Mine too, why on earth would they do that to us?"

I chuckle at the thought now, but at the time, I shared in her frustration, thinking, why indeed would they do that to us? I now realize the more important question that she and I should have been asking was, who told you to eat them?

If you are in the same frustrating situation in which others are bringing "temptations" into your presence, then ask yourself the question that we sometimes fail to ask: Who is giving me permission to eat it? The answer to the question is the person who is responsible for your behavior. No one made me eat the ice cream cake; I was responsible for my own behavior, and so are you.

Just because someone brings something that you desire into your presence doesn't mean that you have permission to actually eat it. Unless you are reading this book in prison, then *you* are the only person who can give yourself permission to do anything.

The more you take accountability for your actions, the more you will feel empowered for in those actions. In the future, when you are having feelings of regret, and wonder why you ate something, speak the answer out loud. Speak life to your words by knowing that you are being held accountable to yourself. Hold yourself accountable by knowing that you are responsible for answering to you.

Being accountable for your behavior will have a huge impact on the choices that you will make in the future. It will minimize the excuses you will make for yourself when you are tempted to veer off course.

Recently, while chatting with a friend about her weight-loss experiences, I began to pay close attention to the excuses for her slow progression. I casually asked her how things were going. At first she blamed her setbacks on her busy schedule. On another occasion she blamed it on family issues. On another occasion she blamed it on being too tired, stating that she was just grabbing things on the go. When you lack true accountability for your actions, you will find yourself going nowhere fast.

In my opinion, there is a sense of pride that comes with holding yourself accountable. Knowing that you are the only person who is responsible for your *results* also means that you are also the only person responsible for your *choices*. You can have other mates on the journey with you, but you will be held responsible as the captain. What does this mean? It means that if the ship sinks, you better still be on it; do not jump ship ahead of time. You are the captain on this journey, and you will need to make the right choices to keep the ship afloat. Believe in yourself and your abilities to stay afloat and you will not sink the ship.

There will be times when others will want to steer the ship for you, but please do not allow them to do so. Sometimes those who love us want us to lose weight and maintain a healthy diet far more than we want it for ourselves.

Make sure that no one wants the best outcome for you more than you do. I personally have been guilty of this, and it didn't help the person whom I so desperately wanted to help one bit. If anything, when others want more for us than we want for ourselves, it can sometimes hinder our growth.

In 2004, several of my family members flew from North Carolina to Houston to attend my wedding. When I arrived at the hotel I could not believe my eyes when I saw one of my aunts. She had gained so much weight that I barely recognized her; it seemed surreal to me. In only six months she had gained so much that she had become what most would classify as morbidly obese. I was very concerned for her health; I desperately wanted to do something to help her lose weight.

During my big wedding weekend, I can recall having a conversation with my mother, asking, "How could you allow her to get so big?" My mother looked at me with disappointment on her face; her only response was, "I have tried to do something about it, we all have." Everyone was attempting to make themselves accountable for my aunt's weight gain—everyone, that is, but my aunt.

Although walking had obviously become difficult, it did not affect my aunt enough to want to change her behavior. The first day after she arrived in Houston, she went out for dinner and ate a fisherman's platter—all items fried. When I spoke to her the next morning she was inquiring as to where she could find a breakfast buffet; my heart sank. It was clear to me and everyone else that food was an obsession for my aunt.

During one conversation that weekend, I gently asked her if she should eat as much as she was eating. She told me no, and joked that she had needed two seats on the airplane on her flight to Houston. Although she made it appear as a joke, I sadly realized that it was actually the truth. I noticed my aunt would casually make fun of her weight to try to avoid the obvious, which was that she desperately needed to lose some of it.

After my wedding, I was on a mission to help my aunt lose weight. I talked to her every single day, trying to determine ways to help her to accomplish some form of weight loss. I would offer suggestions that she wouldn't follow through on, and I would give her techniques to apply to her life that she would completely ignore.

She failed to take any accountability for her eating behavior; she simply ate whatever she felt like eating.

By not holding herself personally accountable she was allowing herself to avoid taking any action about her weight problem. As time passed, I would get frustrated with my aunt and her lack of commitment to bring about much needed changes in her diet. In return, she would get frustrated with me for constantly insisting she actually do something about her problem.

I now understand that my aunt's frustrations stemmed more from wanting to do something and not actually knowing what to do than anything else. I now can understand from firsthand experience the sense of helplessness that she must have been feeling. In addition to that, with her lack of accountability she was unable to justify the need to take any action to change her eating behavior.

In 2006, my aunt was diagnosed with cancer; her obesity was a major contributing factor. Several complications arose during my aunt's cancer treatment as a result of her obesity. It was indeed a tough battle for her, and within seven months she lost that battle.

In her final days, my aunt accepted and acknowledged that her weight problem had played a major role in the deterioration of her health. Although she was aware of the consequences of being overweight, she never beat herself up about her choices. I believe that my aunt would have made different choices if she had known the true risks of being overweight. My aunt and I talked every day during the final days of her life. Although she never shared any remorse about her overindulgence in food, I knew deep down inside she had regrets.

In retrospect, I don't believe my aunt was knowledgeable on the ramifications of being overweight, let alone being morbidly obese. I am sure that if she was more educated on the impact of obesity on her health she would have taken measures to get her weight under control. When my aunt died, she left her thirteen-year-old daughter without a mother. I am sure if she knew what consequences her actions would have produced she would have made different choices along the way.

Unfortunately, in life, hindsight is 20/20. And some life lessons are learned a little too late for those who learn them. For some people, the lessons that are learned by others can be used to their benefit. Experience by far is the slowest way to learn a lesson. If your health is at risk because of a weight problem, please know that it is not too late to make changes to improve your health. You can start today, and the first step is to begin by holding yourself accountable.

Being proactive with your health is very important; you need to make a commitment to yourself that you are the only person responsible, you are the captain on this journey. Hold yourself accountable for your results; don't allow others to want more for you than you want for yourself. Don't expect others to do more for you than you do for yourself. Keep in mind that it's a great idea to enlist support from others to have as accountability partners, but this journey is yours and yours alone. Commit to fully owning it and being one hundred percent accountable for your success. I believe in you and your ability to be accountable!

CHAPTER 11

Patting Yourself on the Back

For me, the beginning of my lifelong journey began soon after I gave birth to Jayda. During pregnancy I was labeled as an "excessive weight gainer" by my doctor. No one likes labels, including me. As soon as I delivered Jayda, I intended to shed the label. I was determined to get the weight off.

I despised the label. Each time I went to the doctor, his voice echoed in my head. I could hear the words ringing whenever he said it: *excessive weight gainer*. I heard it over and over again. During my pregnancy, I was determined to prove the doctor wrong. I wanted to prove that I could control my weight gain during pregnancy. With each doctor's visit, I committed to changes in my eating behavior. I wasn't trying to lose weight, but I did need to get the rate at which I was gaining it under control.

One month, I selected one thing to eat for lunch, and I consistently ate the same thing every single day. My lunch consisted of one scoop of chicken salad on a bed of lettuce, accompanied by a side of fresh fruit.

Weeks later, when it was time for my next doctor's visit, I felt a great sense of accomplishment. I felt I had finally gotten a handle on my rapid weight gain and was eating healthier. I walked into the doctor's office with great confidence. I stepped onto the scale, feel-ing secure.

Before I could clearly focus my eyes to see the numbers on the scale the doctor asked, "What on earth have you been eating?" Then he jokingly asked, "Do I need to wire your mouth shut?"

I couldn't believe it, but there it was, my truth—the scale does not lie. I had gained twenty pounds in one month. I began to plead my case to the doctor, explaining how I changed my diet to a healthier one. I told him that I just didn't understand how that much weight gain had occurred so quickly.

The doctor listened intently, and then he interjected, "It was the fruit." I thought to myself, *the fruit*, and then he said, "Yes, the fruit; it metabolizes into sugar." My heart sank, as did my confidence level. There I sat with a twenty extra pounds, feeling even more over-whelmed than I had felt before. I was extremely discouraged at that point; I had no idea how to slow my weight gain.

When I left the doctor's office, I was determined to take deliber-ate and consistent action to change my eating behavior. I pledged that day that it would be the last day I would be surprised when I stepped on a scale. As time passed, my declaration proved to be correct, and I gained only seven pounds over the last four months of my pregnancy.

Although I was able to change my behavior, I was still faced with one serious problem. I weighed over two hundred and seven pounds; unfortunately, the damage had already been done. My spirit was crushed.

After giving birth, I was still tittering at the two hundred pound mark; the weight remained even after the baby arrived. I didn't know where to begin to get the weight off. In retrospect, I now realize that my defeated spirit contributed to low self-confidence, which greatly impeded my progress. The feeling of defeat fostered a sense of failure in me.

Initially, I did not begin the journey from a good starting place. I didn't know the importance of starting well and the impact it would have on my progress. Self-doubt is a hindrance to your upcoming success. If you don't think you can do something, more often than not you won't be able to do it.

On most days, the weight was all I could think about. My obsession with wanting to lose weight began to affect my mood as well as my attitude, and before long I found myself stuck in a rut.

Perhaps you are wondering, if I could go back in time what would I have done differently? The answer today is simple. I would have helped myself by simply giving myself a break. The bottom line is I went from gaining twenty pounds in one month to only gaining seven pounds in four months. I should have never weighed myself down with feelings of self-doubt. Instead, I should have been patting myself on the back for the enormous decrease in the rate of my weight gain, but I wasn't. I was doing quite the opposite.

Why is it so hard for us to pat ourselves on the back when the progress that we see is not as great as we had hoped for? Why do we ignore our victories because we consider them to be too small to celebrate? I have been guilty of this numerous times. Instead of acknowledging small progress I would ignore it altogether, lowering my confidence. The low confidence level always worked to decrease my expectations for future success.

If this is you, too, then commit to changing this way of thinking right now. It is more than OK to pat yourself on the back for any progress that you make along your journey. By embracing all successes, big as well as small, you then will increase your level of optimism. Try to avoid feelings of self-doubt and disappointment by celebrating successes no matter how small you consider them to be.

If you lose two pounds when you had hoped for seven, then encourage yourself to celebrate anyway. Celebrate that you *lost* two pounds instead of *gaining* two pounds! In the periods that you don't lose anything, learn to celebrate that too! Every accomplishment that you make is a cause for celebration. It's just as important to learn to celebrate not gaining weight as it is to celebrate losing it.

My mood, attitude, and progress all were impacted by my ability to celebrate small successes. My confidence level began to soar with each small celebration. How many times have you stepped on the scale and realized that you have lost two, three, four, or five pounds or even more? When you see small results do you find that you are allowing yourself to be consumed with positive thoughts of accomplishments or negative thoughts of failure?

If this is you, start allowing yourself to celebrate your victories, no matter how small you consider them to be. A small victory is still a victory, and it should be celebrated.

When I interviewed Stella, she shared with me that she had lost seven pounds in twenty-one days. When I asked if she had celebrated her successes, she hesitated. She said, "It was only seven pounds, that's too small to celebrate."

She confessed that she didn't feel the desire to celebrate what she considered such a small victory. I asked her if she was fully aware of how great an accomplishment losing seven pounds is. Initially, she said she was excited about the loss but that others around her appeared to not notice any change in her appearance. I understood that Stella may have wanted others to celebrate her success, but sometimes it is just not reasonable to expect them to do so.

Honestly, others may notice your progress or they may not. The point is, you cannot rely on the opinion of others to increase your confidence or self-esteem. The most important opinion that you should ever care about is your own.

What do I mean by this? If you know you have been sacrificing and working hard but don't get affirmation from others, then don't worry. You have permission to pat yourself on the back. I encourage you one hundred percent to pat yourself on the back for any and all accomplishments that you achieve!

When you are making progress, then look in the mirror and mentally throw your own ticker-tape parade to celebrate. You will have worked hard to earn the right to celebrate any successes, no matter how small you may consider them to be.

Now, I hate to be the bearer of bad news, but sometimes people—yes, even friends—for whatever reason won't acknowledge your weight loss successes. In some instances, people—yes, even friends—may be very critical when it comes to the weight loss success of others. This especially may hold true if these people are attempting to lose weight themselves.

This behavior can be attributed to human nature. It's simply how human beings sometimes behave. The good news is that this behavior has nothing to do with you. I believe this type of behavior stems from the insecurities deep within others. My point is, don't allow yourself to rely on others for a pat on the back. If you do, you may never receive it.

Learning to celebrate *you* and patting yourself on the back does not make you a bad person. Learn to encourage yourself; even if no one else is there to say so, you have definitely earned the recognition.

I have personally experienced how it feels when those around you don't acknowledge or celebrate in your weight loss successes.

My experience in this area was connected to my first pair of skinny jeans. I made the purchase a year after giving birth. I was invited by a group of friends out to dinner; the special occasion was my birthday weekend. It had been months since I had joined my friends for an outing, mainly due to how uncomfortable I felt about my appearance. It had been months since I had seen any of them. To honor the occasion, I decided to treat myself to a new pair of jeans.

Out of fear I refrained from shopping for months—many months. I was not even aware of my actual jean size. I started with what seemed reasonable, a misses' size 6. The fit was not quite right. It was too large. I thought to myself, this is a good sign. I decided to try my luck in the junior department. I selected a size seven but even this was too large. With a huge smile on my face, I rummaged the racks for a junior size four.

I held the jeans high in the air in front of me. They looked so tiny to me. I thought there was no way I could actually fit into them. Without further hesitation I tried the jeans on and, to my surprise, they fit perfectly. I smiled, and rushed directly to the register to finalize the purchase. It was my first pair of skinny jeans, and I couldn't have been more elated.

I was so proud of myself. I rushed home to prepare for the evening. I was so excited and anxious about my new skinny jeans that I arrived to the venue ahead of schedule. I was so early that I unfortunately didn't have the opportunity to make a grand entrance. I was already seated when everyone else arrived.

After dinner we decided to move the birthday celebration to another venue. Throughout the evening I was imagining how great I must have been looking in my new skinny jeans. My self-confidence was at an all-time high. I was one year older and I was wearing the tiniest jeans that I had ever worn in my life.

While my friends and I were standing around enjoying the second part of the evening, I caught a glimpse on the face on one of my friends. She was staring at me, with a look of disgust on her face. Out of sheer concern, I asked her if there was a problem. She frowned at me and said, "Oh my God, I haven't been that skinny since high school."

I could not believe it. I immediately thought, could she possibly be "hating on me" for being thinner? There I stood, faced with a harsh reality. Within a split second my friend had single-handedly deflated my self-confidence. I continued to smile, and shrugged her comment off, but inside I was deeply hurt.

I know you are thinking, why would a friend do something so hurtful to another friend? Well, all I can tell you is that my friend was very much overweight. She struggled with losing her post pregnancy weight for more than ten years. You would think surely of all people she would have been the first to celebrate in my success. Of all the people who truly didn't understand the struggle, she wasn't one of them. You would think that, having lived through the struggle for more than ten years herself, she would be supportive. In fact, she wasn't supportive at all.

My friend was actively in the weight loss struggle on a daily basis. I knew firsthand how difficult losing weight had been for her. I also was aware that my friend was aware that pregnancy weight was just as difficult to lose as any other type of weight. She and I both knew that it didn't matter if you had been carrying the weight for one year or ten years. Weight, regardless of its origin, is still difficult to lose. It doesn't matter how you gain weight, once you gain it the weight belongs to you. I thought my friend would applaud my success and not criticize it. Unfortunately, she didn't share in my victory over conquering weight issues; instead she attempted to shame me for my weight loss.

I didn't understand why my friend had done this to me until one night I was out to dinner with my mother. During dinner that evening, I complimented my server on her sleek appearance; she looked amazing. My server thanked me; then she went on to tell me how much she appreciated the compliment. She told me that her friends had crumbled her self-confidence by insulting her appearance by consistently telling her that she was too thin. I was puzzled, I asked her why would someone tell her that, when she looked so good? She shrugged her shoulders, she having no answer at first.

But then she told me that she suspected that she was a victim of "skinny-shaming," and it had lowered her confidence and deflated her self-esteem. Afterward, I did some research on the topic to sadly learn that some people will make others who are thin feel ashamed about it. I then better understood my friend's comment regarding my skinny jeans. Her comment had nothing to do with me and everything to do with her own insecurities.

So what do you do if this happens to you? You refuse to allow others to project their insecurities onto you, and you go ahead and celebrate your successes! Be proud of your results even if others do not share in your joy.

Remember, beliefs affect thoughts, and thoughts affect feelings; and all of this determines an individual's behavior. This is the reason that it is extremely important to only focus on what you believe and how feel about yourself. Do not allow the opinions of others to affect you or your thoughts and beliefs. The bottom line is that when it comes to you, the only opinion that counts is your own.

The way you actually gained weight has no impact or influence on how successful you will be at losing it. Two hundred thirty pounds is two hundred thirty pounds, regardless if you have carried it thirty days or thirty months—or thirty years, for that matter. How you gained your weight doesn't make losing it any easier.

There may be many roads that have lead you to where you currently are. My goal is to help you to maneuver from where you are regardless of how you arrived here. The ultimate goal is to arrive at a place where you are able to gracefully move forward toward your destination. Be sure to celebrate yourself every step of the way.

Losing weight can sometimes feel like an upward battle, and that can cause a decrease in your self-confidence. Because of this it is imperative to your own well-being to learn to pat yourself on the back. Patting yourself on the back will lift your spirit even when others are doing things to lower it. Do not allow the opinions of others to affect you, lest you find yourself in another pitfall. If this is the case, you will feel as though you were shoved there as opposed to falling there.

Now, don't get me wrong; by no means am I saying go around town tooting your own horn with flags waving your own weight loss successes and accomplishments. What I am saying is to acknowledge when you are making progress, as others may be reluctant to do so.

As you move forward hitting your milestones and targets, acknowledge where you are, embrace it, and celebrate it. Your successes are worth the glory that you have worked so diligently to obtain. Be careful to never ignore any of your accomplishments, whether they are small or great.

So how do you celebrate your own weight loss success without annoying others? Well, the answer is simple. You don't need to share your accomplishments with anyone else; but you do need to acknowledge your successes, even if you do so silently. Reaching a milestone is important, as it moves you closer and closer to the ultimate goal you aspire to achieve.

As you begin to reach your goals, practice engaging in celebratory activities that allow you to acknowledge your victories. If you avoid a pitfall, celebrate that. If you lose two pounds or don't *gain* any pounds in one month, then celebrate that.

You may ask what the best way to celebrate a success. This is a great question. If you are using food to reward yourself then vow to stop this today. Instead, take a day off from cleaning a room in the house that you are dreading cleaning. Treat yourself to a massage. If you can afford to reward yourself with something that you have really wanted to buy for yourself, then buy it. Be creative in finding ways to reward yourself.

The reward doesn't have to involve spending money. You may want to consider doing some community volunteer work as a reward. After all, there is nothing more rewarding than helping and giving to others!

Reward yourself for successes, but make sure the reward does not relate to enjoying food. By beginning to change your relationship with food you must be mindful that food should no longer be viewed as a reward. If you are guilty of using food as a reward, then revisit the challenges in chapter 6. If you have used food in the past to reward good behavior, practice selecting other rewards. Rewarding yourself for good behavior should no longer have a relationship with food.

As you celebrate your successes, you will experience an enormous increase in your confidence level. Even if no one else celebrates you, then give yourself permission to celebrate yourself. Embrace believing in yourself as encouragement to produce the results than you have never imagined possible.

To help increase your confidence level, use the chart below to identify goals that you don't really believe you can achieve. Add your goals to the confidence-building chart. These goals don't necessarily need to pertain to losing weight. The objective is to increase your confidence in your abilities—period. This concept can be applied to any area of your life.

Achieving goals that you feel are impossible will give a huge boost to your confidence level. Confidence is greatly fueled by having the ability to do things that you don't actually believe that you can do. As you achieve each goal, add the date on which the goal was met as well as how you felt. Once you accomplish the goal then you have permission to celebrate it—you have earned it! Add as many goals as you need so that you can lift yourself to a level of feeling that you can do anything you set your mind to! The feeling of success will propel your confidence to a brand new level. You have worked hard to earn the recognition, so embrace the celebration!

Confidence Building

Target Goal	Date Goal Achieved	How Success Feels

CHAPTER 12

The Motivating Factor

While writing this book, I had the opportunity to interview some extremely fascinating people. I was able to receive insight on weight loss from several highly motivated individuals. Many of the interviewees indicated they were sick and tired of struggling with weight and wanted a lasting solution once and for all. Each person was determined to take action to get the weight off and to keep it off permanently.

During the interviews, I became aware that no two people were motivated by the same things. This indicated to me that no two people would travel the same weight loss journey. I began each interview by posing the same question to each person: "What's in it for you?"

I asked all the interviewees to be open and transparent in their responses. The responses that I received were very candid, as each person exposed his or her most intimate reasons for wanting to lose weight. I soon realized that the answer to the "What's in it for you?" question is the fuel that drives each person's motivation.

The responses that I received covered a very wide range. For some the benefit stemmed from a desire to look better. Some people wanted the benefit of getting healthier to feel better. Then there were some who were battling health issues, and the desire was to improve their current level of health.

One of the interviewees wasn't even fully aware of the benefits that she would receive; she simply stated, "The doctor told me to do it." So she was committed to being obedient to the instruction that her doctor had given. Another interviewee shared with me that she was tired of being tired and she wanted to increase her energy level.

The reasons that were given were all different; one person told me that her motivation was to be able to get off blood pressure medication. Another shared that she was preparing for a family reunion and wanted to be able to turn heads. I was intrigued by the various things that motivated different people. The reasons that were given were all legitimate, and each one made complete sense to me. The bottom line was that no matter what the reason was for someone wanting to lose weight, the benefits to eating healthier were many.

Of all of the responses that I received, there was one that intrigued me a great deal, and I wanted to know more. I began to ask additional questions to grasp a better understanding of the real motivation that was pushing this interviewee to lose weight. Her motivation level was extremely high.

Her name was Stella (we met her before in chapter 8), and she was on a mission to shed the weight once and for all. The interview lasted more than two hours as she shared very vivid details with me as to how she has struggled with weight for the majority of her life. Stella is not new to taking this journey by any means; see she has been on it for over forty years. Stella's weight struggles began at the age of sixteen and have continued to trouble her for the majority of her life.

She told me that one summer day while visiting family out of town, she was resting and heard voices nearby. She heard her sister say, "Oh my God, do you see how fat Stella has gotten?" Stella said the words pierced directly through her heart, traveling to the core of her self-image and shattering it.

Stella couldn't believe her sister was discussing something so personal about her with someone whom she considered an outsider, her sister's male companion, but she never allowed her sister to know that she had overheard her. Stella was mortified, to say the least. On the outside she held her silence, but on the inside she was screaming. She returned home with a crushed spirit.

After that summer visit, Stella's self-esteem was at an all-time low. She knew she was overweight, and she surely didn't need anyone pointing it out to her. She felt that somehow hearing how "fat" she had become out loud made it far more real to her. She was disgusted with her truth. Being overweight affected how she viewed herself as well as how she viewed the perception of others. These feelings lead her to slowly lose all confidence in herself. She began to feel invisible, and her social life suffered badly.

Throughout high school, she was being weighed down by feelings of self-doubt and self-defeat. These types of feelings unfortunately weigh you down even more than physical weight. After high school she met the love of her life and got married. Her motivation to lose weight kicked in at turbo speed, and she was successful in shedding forty pounds within a few short months. By the time of her wedding day she had reached her ultimate goal. It was one of the happiest times in her life. Her self-esteem soared, and it was obvious in the way she presented herself to the world. Her image had gone through a total makeover, and she felt like a brand new woman, one whose head was held high and who knew she was capable of succeeding.

Stella was feeling and looking great, and that reflected in her self-image. She began to put more effort into her appearance and gradually she was able to shift her attitude upward in a positive direction. She was successful in maintaining her weight consistently for three full years. However, her weight struggles returned when she decided to get pregnant. During her first pregnancy she gained forty-five pounds and at delivery she was tipping the scale at one hundred and eighty-five pounds.

She knew she had successfully lost weight before, so she wasn't completely distraught about the extra weight after she gave birth. Having a positive attitude about losing the weight helped her to successfully shed forty-five pounds within a few months. She quickly returned to her pre-pregnancy weight of one hundred and forty pounds.

One year later, after deciding to have another child, the weight gain problem resurfaced. This time she gained more than sixty pounds. At delivery, she weighed over two hundred pounds. Once again, the emotions that she experienced forced her to revisit feelings from her past and she found herself depressed about the weight gain.

Stella shared with me that after giving birth to her second child she was not as resilient as before in getting the weight off. Her weight became stagnant at one hundred and seventy-five pounds. Eventually, her weight began to gradually climb back up, and when it hit the two hundred pound mark this time she knew she needed to do something fast.

Being aware that her weight control had been a constant struggle for her throughout life, she knew she needed to enlist some outside help. Her doctor suggested she join a facility called the Diet Center, and although it was extremely costly, she complied with the doctor's recommendation. She felt she had no choice; her weight was affecting her overall health. She knew that she needed to lose weight and lose it fast.

While participating in the Diet Center program, she quickly began to shed the weight. She lost a total of thirty pounds right away. When I asked her how she was able to shed the weight so fast, she gave me several answers. She first began to tell me how the Diet Center provided her with a plan for changing her eating habits to healthier habits. She went on to tell me how the Diet Center helped her to become more knowledgeable on portion control.

All of a sudden, midstream in her thoughts, she stopped speaking as though she were in deep thought. Then she said to me, "Please, no judging, the real reason was my counselor. My counselor scared the hell out of me." The counselor actually frightened her so much that the fear became the source of her motivation. I would imagine that was one scary counselor to motivate someone to lose that much weight, as we all know that weight loss is not so easy to do.

Her counselor was strict, demanding that everyone follow the rules with no exceptions. In the event that Stella got off track, there would be consequences. She honestly didn't want to have to deal with the consequences of having to confront her counselor if she was not in compliance with the demands that were placed on her. She said that whatever she needed to do so stay focused and remain on track she was committed to doing.

She was responsible for calling her counselor every day and reporting all of her food intake for that day. She said her counselor was extremely harsh on her when she didn't follow her meal plan. On days that she didn't follow her meal plan she knew there would be a confrontation with her counselor at the end of the day.

Confrontation is something that Stella disliked, so she did whatever she could to avoid it at all costs. As I listened, it became apparent to me that the answer to "What's in it for you?" was, for Stella, the desire to avoid confrontation. The fear of the confrontation motivated her to do whatever she needed to do to eat right.

Eventually she ceased attendance at the Diet Center not because of her counselor but more because of the cost to attend. Once she stopped participating in the program, the pounds began to slowly creep back on. She quickly returned to the two hundred pound mark once again.

At the time of our interview, Stella had been on the journey for twenty-one days. Prior to starting, she made a commitment to herself to shed the weight this time. For the first time, she didn't want to do it by way of any quick trendy fad. She vowed this time to do it by way of a healthy lifestyle change. She desired long-term, sustainable results. She was willing to do whatever it took to make that happen.

Twenty-one days into her journey, she successfully shed seven pounds. This was a major milestone indeed. Curiously wondering what could possibly be her motivation after forty-plus years, I asked the question. I asked her, "What's in it for you?" I wanted to know what was fueling her motivation.

After a long pause, she said, "This may sound crazy to you, but the real reason I want to lose weight is to meet a man." When I heard her response, I thought to myself, ooh la la; I wanted to hear more.

I asked why her desire to meet a man motivated her so much. Her response was that men in her age range want a woman who is desirably attractive. To Stella "more desirably attractive" simply translated as *being thinner*. I realized that this is her reality. Each person's reality is personal, and it's not to be questioned or judged. Stella was completely transparent about her desire to lose weight. Each person will have his or her own reasons for being motivated, no one reason being wrong.

This was the first time in Stella's life that she was able to stay on the journey for a long period of time without falling off track. She was winning, and she was doing so without enlisting the help of the Diet Center; she was losing the weight on her own. Stella was progressing far more quickly than she had ever imagined. Her confidence level was reaping the benefits: she was actually believing in herself.

By the time Stella and I concluded the interview she told me her goal is to lose fifty pounds within six months. I have no doubt in her ability to reach and maintain her target weight from this point forward.

You have now seen the importance of avoiding pitfalls as well as finding alternatives to challenges. You also have learned the importance of doing things that you have never believed to be possible in order to increase your level of self-confidence. On your own journey, these things will all be important to exercising intentional behavior in the application of each lesson that you will learn.

By now you may feel as though there is a great deal of work needed on your part to start on your path toward optimal long-term success. You are correct, but there is much in it for you. There will be many rewards.

You will be required to do work. I am certainly aware that no one wants to give up anything without receiving something in return, myself included. Now ask yourself the question, what's in it for me?

Your answer to this question will be the driving force fueling your motivation. You may have only one answer or you may have many. Once you identify the reasons you want to lose weight, then give life to all of your motivators by listing the answers in the next exercise. Your answers will be all of the benefits that you plan to gain by losing weight.

This exercise is to bring self-awareness to the things that motivate you. The answers will reflect your own reality and no one else's; there is no judgment, so be very honest. Stella's motivation is simply to snag a man. Dig deep within yourself; open your mind to discover your motivation and what's in it for you.

Benefit #1 _____

Benefit #2 _____

Benefit #3 _____

Benefit #4 _____

Benefit #5 _____

Benefit #6 _____

Stella was a bit apprehensive to tell me the real reason she wanted to lose weight. She said she initially was tempted to say it was for health reasons. I asked her why, and she said she was a little embarrassed to be so transparent about what was really motivating her.

There are no wrong answers when identifying reasons for wanting to shed weight. Each person is different, and his or her reasons are personal and based on life's experiences.

When I started my journey, my answer to the "What's in it for you?" question was based on my own reality. Allow me to now share some personal insight with regard to one of my past motivators. Four days before I gave birth to Jayda, I weighed in at more than two hundred and seven pounds. I could barely focus on the fact that

I was about to give birth at all. Once I saw the scale go over the two hundred pound mark, my thoughts became consumed with the fact that I was *over* two hundred pounds.

After Jayda was born, I directed my attention to motherhood. Soon afterwards my thoughts reverted back to exactly how big I was. I was completely dissatisfied with my appearance. While nursing Jayda I would sometimes catch a glimpse of my belly bulge and I would feel disgusted. The excessive weight was constantly lurking in the corners of my mind.

These thoughts led me to delay my postpartum visit to the doctor. I simply couldn't bear the thought of stepping on the scale in the doctor's office and hearing the words *two hundred pounds* again. I was hoping to shed as much weight as possible before I returned for my follow-up visit.

When I finally made it into the doctor's office and stepped on the scale, I held my breath. I didn't hit the two hundred pound mark; I was just twenty pounds shy of it. I didn't feel good about myself at all. I began to experience familiar emotions from past times when I had been overweight. My self-esteem and self-image were at an all-time low. I didn't like myself in photos, so I avoided being in pictures as much as possible.

It took me six months to shed the first thirty pounds. So what was my answer to the question, "What's in it for you?" I am more than happy to share. You may be surprised at my answer.

My motivation to lose weight was my husband. After giving birth, my extra weight was at the forefront of my thoughts every single day. I didn't want the weight, and I thought about it all the time. In the evenings, my husband would rub my belly as if he were rubbing the belly of Jolly Ole Saint Nick. Each day I would protest and ask him politely not to do it. I told him that the rubbing of my belly like a genie bottle made me feel even more disgusted with myself. I pleaded with him, but each day he continued to rub my belly with no regard to how it made me feel. He even seemed to get a kick out of it.

Then one day I said, "I refuse to allow this man to make me feel bad about myself." With this one thought alone, I birthed life into my motivation. Each day that my husband continued to rub my belly, the more determined I became to get the weight off. Each rub on my belly fueled my motivation more and more.

After the first thirty pounds were lost, I persevered on to lose more weight. It took another year for me to shed an additional twenty pounds. I didn't rush the weight loss. I took my time and I put more focus on changing my relationship with food than on losing weight.

I did many of the exercises that I have asked of you in this book. These things gradually allowed me to change my mind-set about food. Over time I was able to improve my interaction with food. It's been over six years and I have been successful in maintaining a consistent and healthy weight, never wavering or struggling. I have never restarted the journey; I have simply stayed on track, constantly remaining steady on my journey.

The moral of the story is, it doesn't matter why you want to lose the weight. Initially, your motivation may be about you or it may not be. As you begin achieving your goals, your motivation will become more personal to you. Eventually, your motivation will become all about you, and how you see yourself and how you feel about yourself. After all, who doesn't want to look and feel good about him- or herself?

When I began to see results from all of my efforts, my husband's perception and opinion of me became less and less important.

Although I started the journey initially because I cared about what he thought, in the end I only cared about what I thought of myself.

As I began to see results I received a major boast in my confidence level. Soon my will to achieve my goals soared. Before long, I realized that the only opinion that mattered to me was my own. Over time, my self-esteem experienced a graceful recovery. In the end, I had the utter satisfaction of knowing that I could do anything that I set my mind to. And so can you!

CHAPTER 13

The Road Map to Success

I saved the content of this chapter for last for a specific reason. When traveling, many times people focus on where they want to go, sometimes overlooking the obvious: how to actually get there. It's normal to want to get to your destination as quickly as possible, but it's very important to equip yourself with the right road map for the journey.

Now that you have been equipped with helpful suggestions and practical exercises you are ready for the next steps. This is the beginning of a journey to an unforgettable destination: a new you. Where do you start? At the beginning. To get to any destination when traveling, you will need direction. Once you have ascertained the direction in which you wish to travel, you will need to apply deliberate action to get to where you want to go.

Imagine that you decide to travel, and you know the destination, but the best route to get you there is unknown. As you begin your journey, you decide to look for directions on MapQuest. You take the first directions that are available. Once you have the directions, you are well on your way. You begin making good progress on your travels, but then, all of a sudden, something happens. Halfway into your journey, you find yourself thrown off course by detours, roadblocks, construction, and traffic delays.

The point is that it's best to choose your course wisely, taking into account road conditions that you may encounter up ahead. If not, then you may greatly impact the arrival time at your destination. Just knowing the way to go may simply not be enough.

On the other hand, if you have options to select from you might actually discover there are three or more possible routes that you could take. One route might take longer but be a shorter distance. The next route might be a greater distance but could get you there much sooner. Still another route might allow you to avoid all unknown delays up ahead. Ideally you would want to take the route that allows you the opportunity to avoid delays, as no one enjoys wasting time.

The best route to take on any path is the route that will allow you to get where you want to go in the time that you desire. If you know you need to be somewhere by 5:00 p.m., would you knowingly select a route that doesn't have you arriving at your destination until 7:00 p.m.?

When it comes to your weight loss journey, selecting the right path is important. It's best to follow a path that others have successfully followed ahead of you. You could create a new path for yourself, but why would you want to? A brand new path may contain too many unknown roadblocks that could hinder your success.

For tasks that we know we would like to complete, we generally follow a plan. Six years ago, when I started my journey, I didn't jump in blindly. Prior to getting started I sought the wisdom and counsel of my colleague, Greg, who had already successfully taken the journey that was in front of me.

When I realized that Greg had a plan that produced desirable results, I was pretty sure that plan would do the same for me. When he shared his plan with me, I didn't rewrite it. I simply tweaked what had been proven to work for him, personalizing it to fit my own needs.

Not fully knowing or understanding the "how-to" of weight loss is quite all right. You need a starting point, a road map. The preference should be to choose a plan that has already proven successful for someone else. You want to avoid starting the journey without direction. If you don't have a road map, you risk staying on the journey far too long, and possibly never reaching your desired destination.

In this chapter I will provide to you the road map that I followed on my journey to naturally shed more than ninety pounds. You can modify the road map to make it fit your needs, just as I did when Greg shared his plan with me.

You are more likely to stay on course if you commit to taking ownership of the plan; this will greatly increase your rate of success. Personalizing the road map is important; it will allow you to feel as though the journey is your own and not someone else's.

Remember, the road map should be used as a guideline to get you started. Each person is different; a road map may not work the same for every individual. Use my road map as your starting point, adding personal touches to suit your individual lifestyle. There are several options and variations for you to choose from. Again, it is important to keep in mind that you will be most successful if you customize the road map to suit yourself.

THE ROAD MAP

The road map that I provide here will initially serve as a guide for you to customize to suit your individual needs. In the table that follows, I have given you seven days of customizable menu options to get you started on your journey.

	Monday	Tuesday	Wednesday	Thursday	Friday	Saturday	Sunday
Breakfast	4 scrambled egg whites, 1 slice of Weight Watchers cheddar cheese, 1 low-calorie whole-grain English muffin	1 egg, 2 egg whites, ½ cup low-fat shredded cheddar cheese, ¼ cup diced tomatoes, 1 slice whole-grain toast	4 hard-boiled egg whites, ¾ cup dry oats topped with 1 tablespoon of raisins	1 egg, 2 egg whites, 1 slice Weight Watchers cheddar cheese, 1 low-calorie whole-grain English muffin	1 egg, 2 egg whites, ¼ cup diced tomatoes, 1 cup spinach, 1 slice whole-grain toast	1 omelet containing 4 egg whites, ¼ cup diced tomatoes, 1 cup spinach, 1/2 cup low-fat shredded cheddar cheese	3 scrambled egg whites, 1/4 cup low-fat shredded cheddar cheese, 1 cup spinach, 1 low calorie whole-grain English muffin
AM Snack	1 cup of low-fat yogurt and 1 graham cracker sheet	1 cup low-fat yogurt, 1 cup grapes	1 serving of Special K crackers, 1 wedge of Weight Watchers Swiss cheese	2 granola bars, 1 apple	3 hard-boiled eggs, 1 apple	1 serving 100 calorie pack snack, 1 cup strawberries	1 cup low-fat yogurt, 1 apple
Lunch	4 oz. grilled chicken, 3 oz. sweet potato, 1 cup steamed broccoli, 1 cup strawberries	4 oz. grilled ground turkey burger, grilled onions/peppers, Dijon mustard, thin whole wheat sandwich bun, ½ cup baby carrots, ½ cup celery sticks or ½ celery stick	4 oz. grilled tilapia or salmon, 1 cup steamed broccoli, 1-½ cup cooked brown rice	4 oz. deli turkey, ¼ sliced avocado, 2 romaine lettuce leaves, 2 tomato slices, 2 slices whole wheat bread, 1 cup baby carrots	4 oz. sirloin steak, 4 cups mixed green salad, 3 tablespoons balsamic vinaigrette, 1 orange	4 oz. grilled mahi-mahi, 1 cup steamed veggies, 1 small baked potato	1 large salad with spinach, tomatoes, opinions, cucumbers, ½ cup dried cranberries, 3 tablespoons of raspberry vinaigrette dressing topped with 4 oz. grilled salmon

	PM Snack	Dinner
	1 cup of low-fat yogurt and 1 graham cracker sheet	5 oz. baked salmon, 2 cups steamed spinach, 7 oz. sweet potato
	1 cup low-fat yogurt, 1 cup grapes	5 oz. grilled New York strip steak, ½ cup sautéed mushrooms and onions, ¾ cup cooked brown rice, 1 cup steamed broccoli
	1 serving of Special K crackers, 1 wedge of Weight Watchers Swiss cheese	6 oz. grilled chicken, ¾ cup cooked brown rice, 1 cup steamed asparagus
	2 granola bars, 1 apple	6 oz. grilled tilapia, ¾ cup brown rice, 2 cups steamed spinach
	3 hard-boiled eggs, 1 apple	6 oz. grilled chicken, 4 oz. sweet potato, 1 cup steamed asparagus
	1 cup low-fat yogurt, 1 graham cracker sheet	5 oz. grilled salmon, 1 cup steamed broccoli, 1 small baked potato
	20 baby carrots, 2 tablespoon low-fat ranch dressing	5 oz. grilled mahi-mahi, 1 cup steamed asparagus, 2 cups green salad with 2 tablespoons balsamic vinaigrette dressing

While conducting various interviews for this book, I made an interesting observation: every person made the same comment with regard to knowing what to eat. Each individual told me he or she already knew how to eat healthy. You see, they all knew what to eat, yet they were still struggling to lose the weight.

That was a clear indication to me that although many people may already have a good road map in place they simply don't know how to implement it. My friend, here is where I have come to help you get over this hurdle if you fall into this undesirable category.

How do you successfully implement the road map? Your transformational change will require that you not only follow the road map but also follow the instruction that has been laid out for you in the previous chapters.

Which direction do you go? Let's review our checklist to make sure that we have clear direction on this unforgettable journey. First, you will need to own up to your bad habits. Yes, even the ones that you don't want to let go of. If you want results you will have to take action, and you will have to commit to making intentional and deliberate changes to eliminate bad habits. If you focus on results you will never change, but if you focus on change you will get results. Action brings results! Make a commitment to creating healthier habits; this will allow you to eliminate your bad habits forever. With practice, any bad behavior can be changed into better behavior.

This next recap is a big one. Take ownership and responsibility for *your* journey. This is the only way that you will successfully get to where you want to go. You can't blame others for how you arrived at this place. You also cannot blame others for knocking you off track. If Sally brings cupcakes to the office and begs you to eat one, be responsible. Kindly explain to Sally that you are on a journey and although you appreciate her generosity, you will pass on the cupcakes. This is your personal journey; own it!

To see your way clear on this journey, you will be required to have a good understanding of your triggers and problem areas. It will take some practice to implement alternatives, but you can do it. You will be your own guide in this area. If you know the trigger, you can be on the lookout for it. Do you recall Judith? Once she was aware that change was one of her triggers for unhealthy eating, she was on guard. Judith was empowered to stay on track by being able to counter the trigger with alternatives.

The mind is very powerful. Although this true, you have ability to control the mind by changing your mind-set. Your daily confessions will help renew your thoughts in order to find your motivation. Once you find your motivation, work to stay there. Speak your confessions daily.

Next, you will need to remember to embrace starting small and commit to that. You may want to hit the ground running, but this is one time you want to avoid this way of thinking. You will see the greatest results with slow, steady movement in the right direction. You have learned the importance in recognizing current behavior patterns to make healthy alternatives. This will require sacrifice. I believe in you and in your ability to sacrifice. You can do it!

You identified lifestyle-changing goals in chapter 5. Goals are dreams with a deadline. Your goals give life to the vision of where you desire to go. Your vision gives you direction to get you there. Your success will depend on the daily action that you take. Your ability to remove distractions will greatly increase your success rate.

Next, you will want to focus your attention on establishing life-changing goals. The key is to remember that your goals should be measurable and realistic. Some of them will challenge you; being challenged on the journey is inevitable. Being defeated on the journey is optional.

Make it your priority to commit to success. You may be forced to fight a battle on the journey more than once to win it. The point is that this is an unforgettable journey; *do not give up on you*! Every day that you succeed is one day in which you are closer to achieving your goals.

Next, you will need to practice making sacrifices by placing value on the benefit that the sacrifice will offer. This is a tough balancing act, as no one desires giving up something he or she enjoys. The key is to remember that the end benefit will offer you more value than the sacrifice you are currently making. Remember to start small when making sacrifices and increase your level of sacrifice as you master the balancing act.

The next area that you will need to master is a big one! It is the reason that most weight loss journeys fall off course. It is the *D* word: *discipline*. How do you improve your disciplinary skills? The answer is that you will be required to practice discipline. Remember, discipline is a learned behavior. Spend as much time as you need in this area until you can master it. Many people believe they lack discipline when it comes to food. It is important to remember one key concept: discipline is in the mind, not in the mouth. By changing and controlling your mind-set you have total control over your ability to exercise discipline.

As you better gain control over your ability to exercise discipline, you will also need to work to no longer repeat the mistakes of the past. This may be difficult initially, but as you gain wisdom on your journey the repetition of past mistakes will lessen. If you know that you will eat the blackberry cobbler at Eddie V's Prime Seafood because you can't resist it, then avoid dining at Eddie V's Prime Seafood until your discipline is under control. As I indicated in chapter 6, the secret for people who are able to exercise self-discipline and self-control is that they actually believe in themselves.

You may feel it will be difficult to resist something that you really desire, but it's not. You can change your thoughts to change your behavior patterns. You may *think* you need the blackberry cobbler, but you don't. Practice the exercises in chapter 8 to master the art of changing your thoughts to change your behavior. If you can't act your way to a new way of thinking, then resolve to think your way to a new way of acting. As chapter 8 states, thinking it is believing it!

The next objective is a tough one to master. Chapter 9 identified various pitfalls, but there are so many others not listed that you may encounter. You want to make sure that you can remove any distractions from the journey that will hinder your progress—Sally's cupcakes, for instance. Avoiding and conquering pitfalls will take effort on your part, as well as discipline. Be on guard for the pitfalls, especially that monkey on your back: *sweets!* You will be required to embrace a new friend—*the scale*. It is probably the most honest friend that you will have in your life; the scale will never lie to you. The scale will also help you to monitor and track your progress or lack thereof. You cannot fix a problem if you do not face it.

Next, you will want to make sure that you are fully accountable for the journey by taking ownership of it. I have learned through experience that you cannot lead people to a place they are not ready to venture to. What do I mean by that? I can give you all of the practical exercises, suggestions, and tips, but I can't do the work for you. I can lead you to where you want to go, but you will only get there if you are willing to do the work that is required.

Your next focus should be on celebrating your successes. Success may come quickly or it may not. It may come abundantly or it may not. The important thing to remember is that no success is too small to celebrate, no matter how disappointing it may make you feel. It is important to celebrate the loss of two pounds, even if you were hoping for six. Think of it like this: you could have lost nothing or, even worse, you could have *gained* two pounds! My point is, all victories are worthy of glory. It is very important to celebrate your successes along the journey.

Along those same lines, remember that it is also important to avoid the intake of negative feedback or comments from others who may not have your best interests at heart. Support systems add great value on the journey. I am not suggesting that if someone is saying something that you don't agree with that you ignore him or her. What I am saying is that those in support of your journey will seek to encourage, motivate, and inspire you to achieve your goals. But if feedback from others is not helping you in any way, or if it is negative, then kindly refuse it. You will want to remain positive at all times. You don't want feedback that results in a setback. Support should function as a pillar, not as something weighing you down.

I want you to read this next objective over and over again until you are able to internalize it: *commit to making the commitment.* Many plans fail from a sheer lack of commitment. I can lead you, but I can't do the work for you; it's as simple as that. What are *you* willing to do for *you*? Are you willing to make the commitment to do the work that is required to achieve the results that you desire? If so, quit making excuses. We only make excuses when we wish to avoid making commitments. Remember Candis in chapter 6? It's been several months and she still hasn't returned any of my calls! The key is to remember that knowledge + patience + commitment = success!

The final objective that I will recap is almost as challenging as discipline: finding your motivation. I like to think of it like this: motivation gets you going and discipline is what you do when motivation takes a break. How do you force yourself to get going? What is your motivation? What is the number one reason you desire to lose weight? What are the most important reasons? Allow these reasons to be your focus. Let these reasons—whatever they may be—be your encouragement to get motivated. Let your motivation jump-start your engine to throw yourself into full drive on the journey. Your motivation is very important. If you lack motivation, seek it, get it, and encourage yourself to keep it!

Now that we have recapped all of the checklist items that you will need to master on the journey, I want to address one additional item. Many of us fall into the trap of comparing ourselves to other individuals. Others might be on the journey, they might have already completed it, or they might never even have taken it. It is tempting to compare where you are with where someone else may be, but avoid this trap at all times. You are a unique individual. If you feel that you need to compare yourself to someone, then compare yourself to the person you were yesterday.

Don't allow your current relationship with food to prevent you from having the relationship that you so desperately desire. Winning on this journey requires change, and change comes from within. You are a winner, and you will succeed. Have faith in yourself and refuse to give up on you. You will become what you want to be by consistently being what you want to become each day. You have the power to make the change. The only thing that I am sure of is that anything worth having is worth working for. Winning at anything requires you to make some significant sacrifices.

Know that the changes you need to make will require sacrifice coupled with a change in mind-set. If you continue to progress on the journey without changing how you feel regarding food, then you will lead yourself into a pitfall. Equip yourself to avoid the pitfalls by being more mindful of what you are thinking about food. Changing your mind-set is not an easy task, but it is possible.

So how do you change your mind-set? You have to develop an appreciation for what you stand to gain. What you are gaining has to provide more value to you than what you believe you are giving up. As you maneuver through your journey, you will be faced with challenges and will need to ask yourself, is it worth it? There will be trade-offs as well as payoffs. For situations in which you need to make changes, practice exercising the power that is within your control and just say no!

The road map to your success lies within your reach. No one else is responsible for producing the results that you desire other than you. There is a transition that you need to make; the transition is to go from loving food to liking food. If you can master this, you will experience a huge payoff on the journey.

Ninety-five percent of your success will result from five percent of your effort. Your success depends upon where you are willing to place the most value and importance—on your love for food or your love for self.

How many times have you started on a weight loss journey only to find yourself rationalizing and negotiating to have your cake and eat it too? I have done it myself, but if you want to succeed, then you have to be honest with yourself. Accept that if you actually eat your cake then you can no longer have it to eat later.

Actually, you will still have your cake, but you can only eat it once; you will have it on your hips, your thighs, your stomach, or your rear. There will be choices, decisions, and consequences. Encourage yourself to choose wisely to gain the most benefit and add the most value *for* you and *to* you.

The feeling of deprivation is only present when you feel as though you are missing out on something. This is why it is imperative to you to have a thorough understanding of what you are gaining versus what you are giving up. Being fully aware of what you stand to gain will prevent you from feeling like you are losing anything when you pass up certain types of food that you may think you really desire to eat.

It can be fried chicken, blackberry cobbler, chocolate cake, pecan pie, or (you fill in the blank here). In order to change your current behavior with food, it will require you to change how you think about food.

The only person who knows what you really think about food is you. This means you are the only person who will have the power to bring about change. I can't tell you what to think or how to feel about food. Those thoughts come from within.

Don't get me wrong; it's quite all right to like food, but don't fall in love with it. It's difficult to let go of anything that you believe you may be in love with. Food is no exception. Gaining control over your behavior will also require you to frequently practice the disciplinary techniques in chapter 6. Changing your mind-set is a slow and steady process. The good news is that change will come for you. With a little practice, discipline and self-control, change will be achieved.

Now take a moment to complete one final exercise. I want you to identify what you think about food; then give life to your thoughts by writing them down. The objective is to change your current unproductive thoughts to more positive thoughts. Take your time to come up with realistic and positive responses that reflect your current negative thoughts regarding your behavior toward food. You will next replace the negative thoughts with positive thoughts that will propel you even farther on your journey. Great job, you are doing awesome!

Negative Thought   **Positive Thought**

The following are lifestyle principles that I follow daily to remain on track on my journey. Keep in mind that this is a lifelong commitment, a lifestyle change, so the principles will be lifelong too. The journey does not end once you reach your desired goal. Once you reach your unforgettable destination, you will need to continue moving forward on your journey with consistency. Consistency produces results.

Reaching your goal is not the end; you will need to work to stay there, otherwise you will find yourself starting the journey all over again, perhaps many times. I am sure that you do not want that for yourself, and I don't want that for you either.

Lifestyle Principles Are a Lifelong Commitment

- Engage in physical activity three to five times a week for forty-five minutes to an hour each day.
- Drink plenty of water.
- Eat breakfast, lunch, and dinner; customize your road map with sensible selections.
- When making food choices, make deliberate choices that are healthy.
- Consistent behavior produces consistent results.
- Enjoy one sensible snack between each meal.
- Keep your metabolism churning by having meals and snacks two to three hours apart.
- Don't eat just because you see food; practice and exercise your power to say no.
- Practice discipline and self-control daily.
- Team up with an accountability partner for support, but practice being accountable to yourself.

- Be aware of everything that you put into your mouth (food and drinks); write it all down in a journal and review it daily—it makes you accountable.
- Learn to *like* how you look today and *love* the new you that is on the way.

I am aware there is a lot to digest and take in at this point, but do not feel pressured. You increase your chances of success by starting small. Start where you are, embrace where you are, and take it from there.

You can simply start by adding an extra glass of water in your diet daily. You can start by taking a walk around your neighborhood daily. You can start by replacing junk food with a healthy snack, or you can simply start by saying no to something that you would normally say yes to. Each day, add to your list of goals; soon you will be a soaring goal achiever.

Learn to embrace being comfortable with where you are starting. Being comfortable with where you are will help you to make the changes in your diet that are sustainable over the long run. This will allow you to avoid making quick changes that you will find difficult to maintain.

Changing your lifestyle will require work, but it doesn't need to feel like work. You will know that you are making changes in your lifestyle, but only take on the amount of change that you are actually ready to commit to. As you make changes, you will feel more empowered and in control of your eating habits as well as more in control of yourself.

Your confidence and self-esteem will reap the benefits as you begin to see results. The good news is that you have total control over the results that you will receive. You can start as small as you like, or you can move along the journey a bit more swiftly. I will be traveling alongside you every step of the way, but please remember, you are the captain and you hold the power.

Changing your lifestyle may require you to change other thought patterns that may get in the way of your progress, hindering your growth. Let's recap some key philosophies; feel free to revisit this section if ever you feel discouraged along your journey. Or you can simply revisit it when you feel yourself falling off track.

> Quick weight-loss diets are fads that do not produce long-term results; long-term results take time, so be patient with yourself.
> You can't have your cake and eat it too (actually you *can* have it, just not where you want it).
> You have to give up something to gain something.
> Everything worth having is worth working for.
> Ask yourself, is it worth it? If it's not, practice saying no.
> What's in it for you? Your answer will drive your motivation.
> Start slow to maneuver more gracefully and steadily on your journey.
> Why rush a lifelong commitment? Take your time and choose wisely.
> Changing your long-term eating habits is a lifestyle change; make choices that you can sustain and honor.
> Motivation gets you going and discipline keeps you growing.

As we end and as you begin, I want to share with you some words of encouragement. Being able to encourage yourself will be imperative to your emotional well-being. *Falling* off track is normal; *failing* off track is not. When you fall off track, pick yourself up as gracefully as possible, dust off the cookie crumbs, and get right back on your journey.

When you fall, the bruises will be temporary reminders that you have slipped and fallen. But bruises are not permanent. Falling off track does not give you permission to end the journey; it gives you permission to know that you are human.

You are allowed to make mistakes, but you cannot stay in that same place when mistakes occur. No matter what happens, be encouraged that you will be victorious along your journey. Your success will continuously increase. If you are not winning on the journey, you will simply be learning, but you will never be losing. I have taken this journey, and I was successful, and I believe in you that you have the power to be a winner too!

Know that you are beautifully and wonderfully made. I will be traveling alongside you as you move forward on the road to weight loss success. You will achieve all of your goals by putting consistent and deliberate action behind your thoughts. Very soon you will be looking and feeling the way you were destined to look and feel, and that's sensational. Get ready to rejoice and celebrate in being a winner. You are embarking on an unforgettable journey that will lead you to experience a personal transformation. There is a new you on the other side waiting to be discovered!

25723216R00088

Made in the USA
Charleston, SC
09 January 2014